CW01502237

CONTENTS

INTRODUCTION

Why This Book?

For me, taking care of my health began at an early age. The quest started when I was just 15 years old. This is usually the time when teenagers load up on junk foods and the newest, coolest, highly advertised snacks. I, on the other hand, discovered natural foods and health supplements.

It all began by watching the Merv Griffith show. Tuning into Merv and watching Sandy and Durk Pearson give advice on nutritional products was my introduction into the components of healthy eating and nutritional supplements. I remember that show vividly. Durk and Sandy, a little eccentric in appearance, made complete sense when they talked about natural supplements: feed your body the nutrients it needs through nutritional supplements and help to correct or avoid health issues later.

There was so much to learn about during those early days. Back then computers were not commonplace, so googling for information or researching online was not an option. My learning was the old-fashioned way and required many trips to the library. My mom was happy because the library trips were one of the few places that she would drop me off by myself for a few hours while she ran her errands.

The Vitamin Bible from Earl Mindell literally became *my* bible for good health and wellness. I feverishly read and researched how nutritional supplements worked to help feed your body and I learned what nutrients it may be missing from your diet and lifestyle. Then I practiced good clean eating before it was trendy. I learned to incorporate nutritional supplements, not the typical Flintstone or One-A-Day vitamin that most people had in their homes at the time, but *real* supplements that addressed symptoms of depletion in the body.

Little did I know that all these things—the initial research and learning and then later having the opportunity to speak with doctors, researchers, and other visionaries in the nutrition industry—would contribute to the career that would eventually evolve. Today, after much studying and learning, my husband and I have been consultants in the natural products industry for over 27 years. Our consulting company primarily focuses on health, nutrition, and beauty products that help people achieve and maintain their health.

The motivation to write this book

Having trouble with pooping is something that many people must deal with day to day. It's also a personal issue that has affected many of my family and friends. I have witnessed them struggle with this basic bodily function that should come naturally and effortlessly without stress and anxiety. I have listened to family, friends, and acquaintances talk about their experiences with constipation and how uncomfortable they were. I noticed that after the initial embarrassment and awkwardness of the topic, within a few minutes, it literally drew people into the conversation to discuss their experiences, feelings, and frustrations associated with difficult pooping.

The final reason I decided to write this book came when I happened to catch an episode of *Oprah's Allstars*. The show has experts like Dr. Oz, Dr. Phil, and Suze Orman, who give advice on assorted topics such as health, money, or psychology. I enjoyed watching the show, and one comment that really stuck in my head was from Suze Orman. The discussion was a women's health topic, and Suze Orman mentioned that she took a calcium supplement to help her maintain her bone health, but really, she admitted that it also helped her to go poop. I couldn't believe that she admitted this on national television.

It was then that I realized just how much of a problem going poop normally and regularly is in our modern-day society. It does not matter how successful or well-known you are—if you can't go, it's a big problem, no matter *who* you are or how much you earn. Everyone wants to go regularly and to feel comfortable when they go. It was an *a-ha* moment—I would write a book on this very topic to help people understand that there are other options, besides laxatives and "traditional" methods, to help get your body on track again.

Another Reason Why...

During the writing of this book I discovered that I developed uterine cancer. It was something I did not expect, after all I practiced what I preached about health and wellness. But I was shocked (who wouldn't be) and scared when the doctor called with my biopsy results. Ironically enough, a month earlier I had just gone in for a routine PAP smear; and the usual uneventful results were mailed to me, "everything is fine, nothing to worry about, see you next year" is what the letter reported. I still have that letter; in fact, I keep it in my desk drawer. Even though my results were fine, my doctor sensed something was not right with my continued symptoms and abnormal menstrual cycle and wanted to do a biopsy. I fought her on this and thought it was unnecessary, but she was firm and *made* me do it. Thank goodness she did! The results were uterine/endometrial cancer. Not easily detected from a PAP smear, it is very difficult to detect and find. She quickly referred me to City of Hope, and my team of doctors proceeded to let me know their course of action. They recommended 6 chemotherapy treatments: 3 before surgery, and 3 after, with a complete hysterectomy in between.

Ten months later I was finally pronounced cancer-free by my team of doctors, nurses and lab technicians. But during my time of taking the chemotherapy treatments, there were very difficult days of not feeling so well; that was to be expected. But honestly, one of the worst side effects of chemotherapy that I did not expect was constipation. Not so much from the chemotherapy, but from the medications that went along with it—prescriptions to help ease pain and nausea, and medication to tolerate and prevent allergic reaction to the chemotherapy. I found out quickly that if the pills reduced pain, nausea, stomach acid, or helped to prevent an allergic reaction, they usually caused major constipation.

So, if you are going through chemotherapy or know someone who is, you can do this! It may seem hard right now, and really frightening, but if I can get through it, so can you. You are stronger than you know or realize. Just power through it! Second, please read the chapter on how to deal with chemotherapy constipation. I will give some of my personal tips on what worked for me using supplements instead of traditional laxatives. It's really simple—nothing too complicated or hard. I hope some of the things I had success with will work for you to make the chemotherapy process a little easier for you or your loved one.

CHAPTER 1: BIG CONCERNS FOR GOING #2

In the U.S., going number two is a big concern for many, many people. The amount they spend just to go poop is staggering. It is estimated that more than $500 million dollars is spent every year on laxatives and constipation-related products. Not pooping enough or constipation symptoms account for more than 2.5 million doctor's office visits in North America, which is in addition to the millions that people spend at the drug store and pharmacy. Did you ever notice that when you go to a club store, drug store, grocery store or big box stores the laxatives are on the end cap? And in Costco's case their monthly coupon mailer usually has a "deal" available for some laxative in a convenient economy size 2-pack version, specially priced just for the Costco customer. And of course, the pallet of laxatives is usually conveniently located on an endcap near the registers, so you won't forget to purchase as you are checking out.

We live in a day when constipation is **so** prevalent that the remedy is on our weekly/monthly shopping list and is available in an economy 2-pack, so you don't run out.

Most people don't start out intentionally wanting to take a laxative every day. First it starts out with occasional use when irregularity happens, then it becomes more frequent as the digestive system becomes dependent upon the laxative. As time goes on the individual cannot go poop on their own unless they take a laxative.

There are individuals that have a medical reason why they need to take laxatives and stool softeners daily, because they have a *medical reason* for having to take them.

But there is a better way, a natural approach to addressing constipation and regularity than taking OTC laxatives and stool softeners. This book can be your guide to help you get back to pooping naturally as possible and minimize the need for laxatives. It's an easy and simple guide, that incorporates diet, exercise (nothing too strenuous) and a focus on wellness for your *whole* body, mind and spirit. You will take small baby steps that you can incorporate into your daily routine that can help tremendously with the smallest effort on your part. The goal is to go as naturally as possible. You can do it! Don't try and do *all* of the suggestions at once in this book. Try and incorporate a few topics and suggestions each week and keep adding on, don't give up. It has taken your body many years to get to the point where it has forgotten what to do on its own. You only have to help it remember by gently reminding it what to do.

CHAPTER 2: SOME BASIC POOPING INFO

Did you know?

Constipation occurs more frequently in women, with a female/male ratio ranging from 1.01 to 3.77. Even though constipation is a common problem, only a small percentage of people seek medical care to resolve their constipation issues. [1]

What Does Your Poop Tell You About Your Health?

Plenty—it gives you the "read-out" of what you ingested, as well as other waste materials that need to exit the body to maintain health. Pooping, or lack thereof, can also let you know if there is a problem with food allergies or medical conditions that need to be addressed by a physician.

What is the "Normal" Amount of Times to Poop in a Day?

When it comes to poop there is not a real standard for "normal." Is it "normal" for you? The shape, texture, frequency, and number of times you go in a given day are all very individual. But perhaps the biggest factor to consider is... is there a big change in the way you are going? This is an important clue. If your poop changes markedly and unusually for an extended period of time, it may be time to give your physician a call and have everything checked out to rule out anything serious that may need medical attention. But "normal" is very different for each person. How frequently you go – or don't go, the smell and texture, are unique to each person.

Frequency, or how often you go, seems to be where many are mis-guided. Not everyone poops each and every day. Nor is daily pooping a requirement for good health. Shocking to hear, despite what you may have heard from the laxative commercials about regularity, but for some people, pooping three times a _week_ is their "normal," whereas others can poop 2-3 times a *day*, and that is "normal" for them.

The best consideration is, how do you feel? Does your stomach feel comfortable? Do you feel like you eliminated completely? No intestinal discomfort during or afterwards? No straining when you do go? No pain? No cramping? No excessive gas? And, the most important question, is this the norm for you? Have you always gone every other day? If so, then that is what is "normal" for you. Or you may not be able to answer this question because you are chronically constipated, have been on laxatives for years and don't really know what "normal" is for you.

Diet is also a consideration—if you restrict your calories and consume less food, you may not have to go each day because the less you put into your stomach, the less you are going to poop. Or if you are eating low carb and not incorporating enough vegetables and fiber, this may also affect your pooping schedule and frequency.

What if you have the opposite problem and you are pooping too frequently? For example, you ordinarily go once a day in the morning, and all of a sudden you start going 3 times a day. Take a look at what you are eating or drinking. Have you increased your fiber intake? Have you incorporated more fruits and veggies into your diet? Are you drinking more water? Or did you eat out at a dive restaurant and consume questionable food and have something bacterial going on? These are all factors that can change your pooping schedule and consistency considerably.

The rule with pooping is...there is no real rule. Instead, you should ask yourself, does it feel comfortable after you go? Is it comfortable while you are going? Is it your usual routine? Do you feel like you have eliminated all the poop and have no urge to go more? Do you feel relieved when you go? The answer should be YES! If it does not feel comfortable, then you may want to speak with your doctor or health practitioner to rule out any health issues.

Other factors like water intake, hormonal fluctuation, menopause, medication, if the weather has been hot and you are sweating more, lack of sleep and exercise can make a big difference in your pooping schedule.

---

1. Pinto Sanchez, MI, Bercik, P. . Can J Gastroenterol. 2011 Oct; 25(Suppl B): 11B–15B. doi:

CHAPTER 3: IS MY POOP THE RIGHT SHAPE?

While we all know that our poop does not stay the same shape (i.e. diarrhea or constipation), many people don't know if their poop is a "healthy" shape. Below is a chart that gastroenterologists use as a guideline.

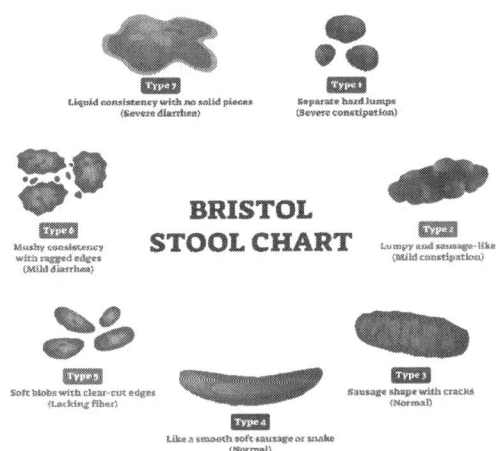

Bristol Stool Chart

The Bristol Stool Scale is a diagnostic medical tool designed to classify human poop into seven categories. It is used as a research tool to evaluate the effectiveness of treatments and diseases in the bowel. It is also one of the tools used in diagnosing irritable bowel syndrome. The chart also gives a guideline for healthy or unhealthy appearance of poop.

The Bristol Chart Explained

Types 1 & 2

If you have hard stools or separated lumps, this indicates constipation. This happens because the large intestine works to remove water from the stool as it passes through the gut. Decreased movement either by problems with the muscles lining the intestines, or by a diet low in fiber lets the poop sit in the large intestine, where more water is drawn out of the poop (dehydrating it), making it harder to poop.

Tip: Eat a diet rich in fiber. You hear that statement a lot. I'm sure your doctor, magazine articles and maybe even your grandma has told you this...but it really does make a difference. Fiber adds bulk and helps your poop to stay hydrated for the entire journey down your intestinal tract.

The average American eats about 15 grams or less of fiber every day.

According to the USDA, that is way below what we really should be eating.[1]

- Women 51 years of age and younger should consume 21–25 grams of fiber daily.
- Men 51 and younger should consume 30–38 grams of fiber daily.
- Women 51 and older should consume 21 grams of fiber.
- Men 51 and older should consume 30 grams daily.

The USDA recommends eating at least 9 servings (2 cups) of fiber-filled fruits and veggies every day. [2] Nine servings sounds like a lot, especially when you are not used to eating a lot of fruit and veggies. But as a note, the serving sizes are not heaping platefuls. They range from eating ½ an orange to ½ cup of fruit or veggies. So, you really won't have to eat tons of fruits and veggies to achieve your fiber goals. The important thing about eating a diet that is rich in fiber is that it helps bulk up the stool, and the fiber acts like a sponge to help retain water, which in turn makes for easier pooping.

If you are not used to eating a lot of fiber, increase your fiber intake gradually, and drink plenty of water to help reduce gas. On a personal note, when I eat foods that notoriously cause gas, like zucchini, broccoli, or beans, I use **Bean-O**®. It is a nutritional supplement that helps you digest gas- inducing foods without experiencing loads of embarrassing stomach noises, cramping, gas pain and the most notorious anti-social behavior - farting. Just take a couple of tablets with water with your first bite, and it magically helps to reduce gas.

Types 3 & 4

This is where we all strive to be. Normal, well formed, easy-going poop. Good job to you all that are 3's and 4's. We will all get there soon to enjoy effortless, perfect pooping like you.

Types 5, 6, 7

When you hear about pooping problems, we mostly think about being con-stipated. But there are many people experiencing diarrhea on a regular basis, up to 75% of the time when they poop. If you have soft, separate, blobby, fluffy pieces with ragged edges or no solid pieces at all, in a kind of a pudding con-sistency, you have diarrhea. Like with constipation, you may need to include more fiber in your diet. It will help to keep your stool at the normal range and less watery.

There are other reasons why you might be experiencing diarrhea, like having bacteria and yeast in the large intestine. Food sensitivities can also cause a myriad of trouble in your digestive system from GERD (gastroesophageal reflux disease) to constipation.

Not Exactly Diarrhea

Consistently soft, pudding-like stools may also indicate celiac disease,which is an inherited autoimmune disease that causes damage to the small intestine when gluten is ingested. Even though many people are going gluten free, in reality celiac disease really only affects about 1 in 100 people (about 1% of the population). About .4% of the population has doctor-diagnosed wheat allergy, according to a 2006 study. In the study group, a true allergic response to wheat, which contains gluten, can include skin, gastrointestinal, and respiratory symptoms.

18 million Americans may have a lesser form of sensitivity that is called "non-celiac gluten sensitivity," which may produce similar symptoms to celiac disease when they consume gluten.[3]

One of the major signs is almost loose pudding-like poop consistently. With celiac disease, the body has a gluten intolerance. Gluten is a protein that is in wheat, rye, and barley. Continued consumption of gluten destroys the villi, the tiny, fingerlike protrusions lining your small intestines, making the body unable to absorb nutrients from the foods you consume. The constant irritation contributes to the loose stools people experience. If you experience this, please consult your physician to schedule a screening for celiac disease. Next, try a gluten-free diet to help your body absorb the nutrition from the foods you eat, to help normalize your pooping, and to help with symptoms like pain, fatigue, bloating, depression, and rashes.

Floaty, Greasy-Looking Poop

Are you eating greasy foods that your body cannot digest? Many people overindulge and feel it in their stomach with indigestion and a soapy feel after eating and later while pooping. But if floaty greasy poop has become more of the way you have been going lately, or maybe you are noticing that there is an oil-slick appearance in the toilet after you go, it may mean your body's ability to absorb fats from food is not occurring. An infection or inflammation in your pancreas may prevent you from producing digestive enzymes.

A food allergy or infection could also be the culprit. It can be damaging to the lining of your intestines that's affecting absorption. Contact your physician for a stool sample test to find out the cause before further irritation and damage occurs.

Stringy or Pencil-Thin Poop

It can be as simple as...you have constipation. But it can also be a symptom of rectal cancer. If you notice pencil-thin poop for a couple of days, usually that is something you don't need to worry about. If you are constipated and straining, it may prevent the muscles in the anal sphincter from opening and can narrow the way your poop comes out. Eating fiber and drinking plenty of water usually helps. Then your poop should return to its normal shape.

But if the stringy or pencil thin poop continues it may indicate rectal cancer. With rectal cancer, the tumor is rigid and fixed, and it encircles the rectum so there's less space for poop to squeeze through, causing the poop to appear thin and pencil-like. Don't wait—make an appointment with your physician for a colonoscopy.

Stress can be a big factor in food digestion and pooping.

Chronic stress and anxiety can take its toll even when digesting foods because of the gut-brain connection.

---

1. U.S. Department of Health and Human Services and the U.S. Department of Agriculture. Dietary Guidelines for Americans. Appendix 7. Nutritional Goals for Age-Sex Groups Based on Dietary Reference Intakes and Dietary Guidelines Recommendations - 2015-2020 Dietary Guidelines. Accessed July 16, 2020.

2. Health.gov. Dietary guidelines. Accessed July 16, 2020

3. Celiac Disease Foundation. 9 things you should know before going gluten-free. Accessed January 27, 2020.

CHAPTER 4: WHAT COLOR SHOULD MY POOP BE?

Simple answer: brown-ish. More expanded answer: the usual color for poop is a shade of brown, but it can reflect what you have eaten as well. If you eat a lot of leafy green veggies, it can look a little greenish/brown. If you eat red fruit or veggies you may see a reddish-brown. Some OTC and prescription medications can alter the color of your poop. Ask your pharmacist about your medications and how it may affect your digestion and pooping if you notice a change. If you have a consistent color change that varies from brown, it is always a good idea to discuss this with your physician.

What Color is Your Poop?

Black-ish Color: If you have taken Pepto Bismol, you probably know that your poop is going to be the color of a charcoal briquette for a couple of days. If you see this, there probably is no cause for alarm, as this OTC medication can cause this side effect. Why does this happen? The reaction occurs when sulfur in your digestive tract combines with the Pepto, and forms bismuth sulfide. The black discoloration is a temporary side effect and is harmless. It may last for several days after you stop taking Pepto Bismol. But it will eventually subside. This is also true if you have taken charcoal capsules or eaten the trendy charcoal ice cream that seems to be popular on social media. Your poop will be black after you eat the charcoal-laden food, and then it should revert back to your usual color in a few days.

Do you take iron supplements? Iron may make your poop turn a black-ish-green shade. But if you haven't consumed any of the above and you have black stools, be careful, because dark-colored stools can indicate bleeding from your upper GI tract that oxidizes as it passes through the intestines. It may also be an indicator of a stomach ulcer. Please consult your physician.

Pale or White Color: Did you take the OTC medication Kaopectate? It can cause pale and light clay-colored stools. If you haven't taken Kaopectate and are experiencing light or white-colored poop, this can also indicate that you may have a more serious problem in your GI tract. Your liver may not be making enough bile due to a blocked duct, tumor, or stone. If bile does not reach the intestines the poop will turn white. This is a common occurrence with diseases like cirrhosis and hepatitis. Please consult a physician if you are experiencing this symptom.

Red Color: Don't immediately freak out! Remember back to what you may have eaten the previous day or so or what beverage you may have consumed. Did you eat something intensely red... like beets? The first time my then boyfriend (now husband) encouraged me to try some of his beet juice, as he was doing a "cleanse" and first thing every morning he would drink beet juice. He offered me some of his juice, I gave it a try and loved it! I had always loved *eating* beets, and I discovered I really enjoyed drinking the juice. But then came the shock of red-tinted pee in the toilet. The red tint comes from a compound called betacyanin in the beets. This color can show up in your pee and poop for a couple of days. So, don't be alarmed if you see a color shift if you've consumed beets or even beet supplements.

If you did not consume beets, then ask yourself if there were some other fruits or veggies that may have caused your poop color to lean towards red, like tomatoes, cranberries, cherries, strawberries, or watermelon. Or did you consume any red dye, like the beautiful red frosting roses on a birthday cake that everyone seems to fight over? The concentrated red food coloring that tints the frosting can show up in your poop and alter its color. So, don't be alarmed if you see the effects later when you poop.

If you did not consume any of the above, you may have blood in your stool, which indicates fresh blood from the intestines. Bright red blood in the stool can indicate hemorrhoids, polyps, inflammation, diverticulitis, or colon cancer. Make a phone call to your physician right away for an appointment. Don't procrastinate or wait for it to get better. Your doctor can help you get the treatment you need before it progresses, as any infection or cancer needs your doctor's care and treatment.

Yellow Color: Yellow poop that floats? You may be having trouble digesting fat, or you may be consuming too much fat in your diet. Many people experience this after gallbladder surgery or other surgery procedures that hinder fat digestion. If you are having a surgical procedure, please inquire with your doctor so you will have a heads up on its impact afterwards.

Yellow poop can also be a result of taking weight loss medications as well. Yellow, greasy, and fatty poop may also point to chronic pancreatitis or celiac disease that needs to be addressed by your physician.

Green Color: Did you eat your Instagram-worthy kale salad today or green drink? That could very well be the reason why your poop is a dark shade of green. In fact, any salad-and greens like spinach or even green beans can cause your poop to drift toward a green shade. Or did you have a few slices of avocado toast? That too can cause your poop to shift to a greener hue.

Did you know that green poop can also be a sign of infection? If your poop is consistently green and it's not food related, then you may have a clostridium difficile (C. diff) infection. It is common and usually occurs after a course of antibiotics. C. diff is a normal part of the flora in your digestive tract. Taking antibiotics can kill off the good bacteria that normally keeps C. diff in check. As a result, the bacteria may proliferate uncontrollably and cause serious stomach issues that can lead to dehydration, hospitalization, and in extreme instances may even be deadly. If you're still taking a course of antibiotics, call your doctor immediately and let them know what you are experiencing

CHAPTER 5: WHY DOES POOP SMELL?

It is normal for poop to have a not so nice odor; it is due to the bacteria in the colon that breaks down food. But if the smell of your poop changes drastically to - extremely bad, and not usual for you, this may indicate an infection. Other health conditions that may cause unusually smelly poop are inflammation of the colon from inflammatory bowel disease and diseases that cause malabsorption in the intestines, like celiac disease, chronic pancreatitis, cystic fibrosis, or even lactose intolerance. If your digestion is healthy most of the processes will take place in your small intestine and you will have some residual of what you ate left in your colon. When you have poor digestion and food sits in the colon for a long time, then bacteria will start to propagate and fermentation proceeds. That's what causes the "bad" smell. If you would like less smelly poop, a diet of more veggies will help give your poop a more neutral odor. If you consume more meat this will increase the smell factor, because putrefying meat does not smell very nice.

Does your poop smell like sulfur or eggs?

Congratulations, you may have giardia. This parasite is found in freshwater ponds or lakes, so if you recently went swimming in a lake or pond, went camping, or drank water from a lake or stream, you may have picked up the bug along the way. You may not notice when or how it occurred. You could have diarrhea for weeks or even months, but otherwise feel fine. Have your doctor run a stool sample test to diagnose and treat with antibiotics to get rid of the pesky parasite.[1]

---

1. Prevention. 7 things your poop says about you. Accessed January 27, 2020

CHAPTER 6: IS THERE A GOOD TIME TO POOP?

Some people have a set schedule for pooping. They have a set routine, like clockwork, and go in the morning. They may drink water or coffee, read for a few minutes, and then go. You can poop at any time during the day, with no set time, but the most common time to poop is in the morning. The caffeine in coffee actually helps to not only get you going in the morning, but also helps to stimulate your bowels to get them going as well.

Experts say that minutes after you ingest the coffee, it makes its way to the stomach and increases the contractions of the gut, which makes you get the "I have to poop" urge as the stool makes its way to the rectum. Caffeinated coffee is the most effective at producing this urge.

There are some biological reasons that you may go in the morning as well. Many people eat their heaviest meal in the evening for dinner. So, when you go to sleep, there have been many hours to let the food digest and move down in the bowels by morning. Most people don't usually wake up to poop, because if you are lying down the bowels close off and you will not "feel" the urge to go until you rise in the morning.

The second most popular time to go poop is when you get home from work. There are a couple of reasons for this. Many people can finally relax enough to go, and the other reason is taking the time to go. It can be difficult if you have deadlines and phone calls to deal with all day long and taking the time to go to work may not be the most relaxing.

CHAPTER 7: WHAT TO DO IF YOU'RE JUST NOT FEELING LIKE POOPING...BUT YOU WANT TO

We've all been there. You have been sitting on the toilet for what seems like an eternity. You've caught up on looking at all of your old catalogs that you've stashed on top of your toilet tank in the bathroom, played a couple of games on your phone, "liked" all of your friends' posts on Facebook and Instagram... and you still cannot go.

Now what?

The puborectalis muscle is what controls fecal continence. Which is the very thing that controls whether you go or not. Did you know that your posture has a great deal of influence on this muscle? It works by looping around the rectum, pulling it forward to create what is called an anorectal angle. This angle determines how easily you are able to go poop.

Our modern-day toilets do not help us create this ideal anorectal angle. In fact, the toilet may put you in the absolute incorrect position to poop easily. Scientific research on this subject shows that when you stand, your colon pushes against the puborectalis muscle. When you sit, this muscle becomes tighter, involving unnecessary tension and strain. It closes off the rectum, making for a difficult time pooping. Straining while pooping can lead to anal fissures and hemorrhoids. [1]

Many doctors recommend that pooping is easier when you squat, instead of the customary 45-degree angle in which most modern toilets position the body. How do I squat and go in my modern toilet, you ask? There are a few devices that are available online and in stores, but the simplest and easiest fix can be a low footstool or a low box that you have around the house. While you are seated on the toilet, put your feet on the footstool or box and it will help to put your body in a position that may help to get things going.

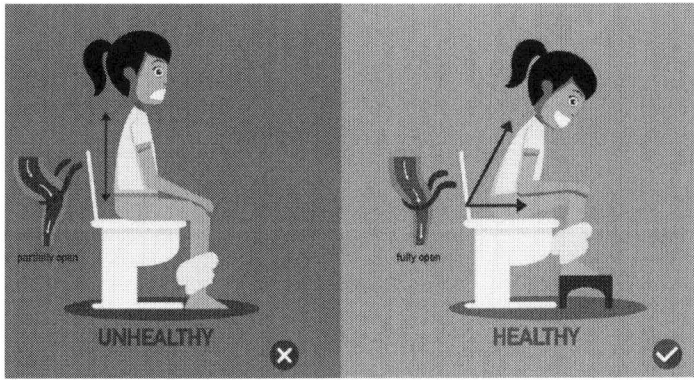

1. Sikirov, D. Comparison of straining during defecation in three positions: results and implications for human health. Dig Dis Sci. 2003 Jul; 48(7): 1201–5. DOI:

CHAPTER 8: POOPING PROBLEMS RIGHT BEFORE AND DURING YOUR PERIOD

Being constipated while you are bloated right before your period is an awful feeling. You kind of feel like a pool toy that is about to burst with PMS bloating and water retention, and when you add the additional feeling of being constipated, well that's just adding insult to injury! But there is a hormonal reason *why* this is happening.

It's all because of the hormone progesterone, which starts to increase between ovulation and when your period arrives. Progesterone can cause your digestion to slow down, so food moves more slowly through your digestive tract. The increase in progesterone also can cause bloating, water retention, headaches, and constipation.

On the opposite end of the spectrum, some ladies experience diarrhea before and during their periods. Another hormone-like substance can cause that reaction in the body— prostaglandins. The endometrial cells produce prostaglandins and are released as the lining of your uterus sheds before and during your period. As prostaglandins increase, they can affect muscles that control your bowels. And just like your period cramps, the intestines also cramp, causing poop to be forced out quickly, causing diarrhea. When period time rolls around, just about every woman knows if she will experience constipation or diarrhea during that time of the month.

Dealing with Period Constipation

In our household constipation before your period seems to be the trend. After years of trying various methods of relieving constipation right before our periods, here are a few tips that have worked for us.

- Upon arising, have some warm water and lemon juice. Just a teaspoon of freshly squeezed lemon juice in 8 ounces of water. If you don't like the taste, add just a dash of honey or maple syrup.
- Drink a cup of coffee. It will help to stimulate your bowels. Most people poop within a few minutes of drinking coffee.
- Increase your fiber intake to include more water-rich vegetables like lettuce, tomatoes, and cucumber. Increase your fiber and water intake in the middle of your cycle, when constipation-prompting progesterone levels start rising.
- Include watermelon, grapes, apples, apricots, tangerines, or oranges into your day. These fruits are high in fiber and water content. Eat at least two servings per day.
- Try eating a hydrating meal that includes vegetable soup. It helps to increase the water and fiber intake and hydrates your digestive tract from

the inside out. Or try some lentil soup, it contains veggies, beans, and broth, and is very filling because of the fiber and will help you go.

- Cut back on white bread, flour tortillas, white rice, pasta products, and cheese. These items can cause constipation and do not contain fiber or hydrate your body.

- Before bedtime try a nutritional supplement called Natural Vitality CALM®. It will help you go poop easier but has the added benefit of giving you the most relaxing wonderful sleep. In our home when our Calm stash starts getting a little low, everyone panics just a little, because it is *that* wonderful to take before bed on multiple levels.

- Most importantly, drink at least 8-10 glasses of water daily to help hydrate your digestive tract.

Dealing with Period Diarrhea

With period diarrhea, it's important to start with proactive measures before your period begins. About 10 days before your expected period, start to implement the following.

- Try taking a psyllium powder like Metamucil, it is a soluble fiber that will help to firm your poop and keep diarrhea in check.

- Take a probiotic supplement.

- Include probiotic foods in your diet like yogurt – if you are lactose intolerant try cashew or non-dairy yogurt, sauerkraut, fermented pickles, or kimchi. Make sure to read the label to ensure that they are fermented.

- Cut down or eliminate coffee during the pre-period time–it stimulates your digestive tract and induces bowel movements.

- Eat more fibrous vegetables, beans, rice, whole grain bread, whole wheat noodles, and if you are not lactose intolerant, cheese.

- Incorporate a 15-20-minute meditation break each day to destress and relax the body and digestive system. YouTube has many mediation videos that are free. Meditation search suggestions: Calming, balancing, chakra balancing meditations. My personal favorites on YouTube are Pure Rasa, Trigram Healing, and Jason Stephenson.

- If you are still having symptoms of diarrhea, you may want to try taking a non-steroidal anti-inflammatory (NSAID). It can block certain enzymes in your body that make prostaglandins. Keeping prostaglandins in check will help alleviate belly ache and diarrhea. Many ladies take 1 tablet/capsule a day a few days before their period and report marked improvement in their diarrhea symptoms. It can also help reduce menstrual cramping. Please check with your physician regarding taking an NSAID.

If period pooping issues become unmanageable, after trying a few of the "natural" alternatives, and please consult your physician. They can help you come up with a plan that will make your period a little more comfortable for you. Pooping at this time of the month should not be annoying, painful, or difficult.

CHAPTER 9:
WHY ARE MEN OBSESSED WITH POOPING AND...WOMEN ARE EMBARRASSED?

Okay...not exactly obsessed...but they seem to have a more no-nonsense attitude towards pooping. You may have noticed that if a man must poop, they just dash to the nearest bathroom, run, and go immediately. Also, when they go, some men seem to stay in the bathroom for what seems like an inordinate amount of time. Am I right? When it's "pooping time," they take books, their cell phones, or even an iPad and stay in there for 20 minutes "pooping.".

In fact, they can close business deals on the phone, while going poop. The best one that I heard was that they are at a "trade show" and they are at the "standard booth" while pooping. "The standard booth" is the manufacturer of the toilet, and the "booth" is the bathroom stall, but in reality, he is just pooping. This is a concept that most women can't even fathom.

It's quite a contrast to women's attitudes when pooping in public. For most, the attitude is closer to "let the anxiety and stress commence." Women will usually procrastinate for hours before we deem it time to go poop. If indeed, things are starting to get "urgent feeling" and we really need to go, then somewhat reluctantly, we will make our journey to the public bathroom to use the toilet.

There are some secrets to using a public toilet for a woman. It is a must use 2-3 toilet seat covers or toilet tissue to ensure that the toilet seat is satisfactorily covered and deemed acceptable to sit on. After all, previous restroom attendees sometimes *do not* stay seated for the entire performance when they are going pee so *they* can avoid sitting on the toilet seat. Thus, they leave quite a mess for those that actually have to sit on the toilet seat to go poop.

As a side note, personally, this was a huge problem when I was going through chemotherapy, and my leg muscles were a little weak from not being strong enough to exercise. I just could not hover over the toilet to pee when it was too dirty to sit on. So, either I had to hold it and go to another location or put down a lot of seat protection. So, for those of you that hover and leave a mess, please be considerate of those that pee after you... we may not be able to hover, so please just use a toilet seat cover. Thank you in advance.

Some women will have a silent "sit-off" until everyone has left the bathroom, so they can poop and not be embarrassed or offensive. Some women, in an office bathroom situation, will lift their feet off the ground so co-workers do not see their shoes to identify the person that is pooping. I highly doubt that anyone would really look to see whose shoes were in "that" stall. But many will even try and <u>not</u> go at all if the bathroom situation is "not right," and just hold it until they get home after work.

Another technique that women will use is to put some toilet paper or a seat cover in the toilet before going to "buffer" any splashing sounds that may occur, so others can't hear what they are doing. There are others that try the "courtesy flush" and keep flushing the toilet so the flushing sound buffers the splashing sounds and gets rid of the smelly poop.

I can remember back when I was dating my then boyfriend, now husband. We had gone on our very first overnight trip together to a mountain cabin. Thinking ahead, I had already strategized that I simply would not poop for a couple of days to avoid embarrassment. I would just not eat a lot, and I would avoid foods that make you go poop. As soon as we arrived at the cabin, he (to my amazement), announced, "Man, I gotta go poop...Nature Calls." He dashed into the bathroom and pooped practically on demand. Well, from that moment on, "nature calls" has been a running joke with us. All shame and apprehension about pooping evaporated in that moment. But many women that are with a new boyfriend will make an excuse to leave and to go to Starbucks or McDonald's just so they can poop in private without Mr. New and Wonderful seeing or smelling them go.

But the true facts are, ladies, we all have to poop—including Mr. New and Wonderful. It is important for women to realize that bodily functions are just fine, and that no one has lavender-mist-scented poop, and that Mr. New and Wonderful will probably not mind one tiny bit if you must poop. And if you have been sneaking around strategizing where and when to go poop, he's probably wondering why you just don't go.

CHAPTER 10: IS STRESS CONTRIBUTING FACTOR IN CONSTIPATION?

Stress absolutely *can* affect the body as it activates the sympathetic nervous system (the fight or flight response), and the body reacts to stress by decreasing bowel movements. After all, pooping in a life or death situation can make you vulnerable.

Many times, when people are in stressful situations, we try to soothe ourselves with comfort foods to help us feel better emotionally. Sometimes those foods aren't exactly the food groups you should be eating from to promote good digestion and pooping. Many indulge in crunchy snacks like potato chips or Doritos, and then follow it up with a pint of ice cream and cookies. Also, many people become sedentary when stressed and drink less water and more alcohol, which of course can cause constipation, dehydrating the body even if you are not stressed out.

If this describes what you may have done or are doing, before resorting to laxatives, try taking a walk, relaxing, breathing deeply, and enjoying the sights while you walk. For some, massage therapy can be helpful—not only is it relaxing, but it can help to drain the lymph system helping you to relax and aid in constipation and induce natural pooping.

Stress management is important for everyone in our hectic world these days. Take a moment to notice if you are feeling anxious. If you are... accept it; don't try to push it away, fight it, or deny your feelings. Accept the feelings. It's okay to acknowledge that you *are* stressed. It sometimes causes more stress to deny than to accept.

Then try to shift your thinking to another positive topic. Think about something that you want to accomplish, or perhaps make a plan to have a relaxing day to yourself, doing all of your favorite things. It will help you regain control of anxious feelings and get past stress. It's okay to feel stressed and anxious, but it is not helpful to replay the stress and anxiety over and over again in your head.

Shifting your mind is a good way to keep from over-thinking stressful situations. It's not something that you will be able to do 100% of the time successfully. But the more you implement this way of dealing with stress, the better you will be able to deal with stress. You will actually retrain your brain to react to stress in a less impactful way. Your aim is to reduce stress, not eliminate it. Keeping stress under control can help to prevent future constipation and help you to live a happier life.

Some Relaxation Techniques to Try:

- Deep breathing—when we are stressed, we tend to breathe shallowly. Meaning, we don't really breathe deeply. This is where just breathing and getting oxygen into the body can help you greatly. When practicing deep breathing, put your right hand on your chest and your left hand on your belly, right below your rib cage. As you take a breath, try to not move the hand on your chest as you inhale. Your left hand on your belly should rise as you inhale. Then exhale slowly and let the air out until it feels like your abdomen touches your spine. Do this 3-4 times and relax.

• Visualization—imagine a peaceful meadow complete with flowers, white puffy clouds, and a meandering stream. Or maybe you prefer an ocean scene with the water lapping up against your sandy toes, or maybe just a lit candle is all you need. Think of whatever makes you feel relaxed without inducing an emotional response from your brain.

• Take a comfortably warm bath with 1/2 cup of Epsom salts to help relieve stress and to help with constipation. Fill the bathtub with warm water and add 1/2 cup of Epsom salts to the water. Stir the water before you enter the bath to ensure that the salts are thoroughly dissolved, and then test the water to make sure it's not too hot for you. You may also want to add a few drops of essential oils like lavender or rose oil. I usually add 20-30 drops, but you can adjust this to your preference. Then relax for 15-20 minutes in the bath. While you are relaxing, your body will absorb the magnesium from the salts through your skin.

The Epsom salts are both relaxing muscles and easing tension, as well as helping to promote easier pooping. I also tend to include a nice glass of red or white wine, because it relaxes me, and the fermented wine in small amounts *can* be helpful in getting your system going. Keep it to one glass though. If you don't drink alcohol, try a cup of chamomile or linden tea, or mineral water with a splash of fruit juice to make it fun and indulgent. I recommend 1-ounce of fruit juice with a natural mineral water and a couple of ice cubes. Juice suggestions: peach, strawberry, pineapple, or whatever you prefer. Just keep the juice amount to 1 ounce.

- Listening to music—for me, music can really shift my mood. If I am feeling a bit stressed, I usually pop on my headphones and listen to music. Tune into music that is relaxing, positive, and fun. Try listening to classical music even if it is not the music genre you normally listen to. Try Debussy, Mozart, or Beethoven. It will relax you and give you a new appreciation for classical music.

- Singing to music—If you haven't been singing in the car lately, maybe you should go for a drive and put on music that makes you want to sing. Did you know that vocalization helps to reduce stress and anxiety? It actually changes your brain chemistry when you listen to music, and when you sing out loud it helps to release endorphins that make you feel better. So, put on your favorite song and sing along like you did when you were a kid.

- Dancing, yoga and stretching—I always remember the saying "a body in motion stays in motion." Keeping your body in motion helps your body stay active, flexible, and vibrant. Fit abdominal muscles help the stomach do their job to keep your posture and organs in the correct alignment and will help you to poop. As with the above suggestion of listening to music, moving and dancing to music is definitely helpful in lifting your mood.

- Meditation—there are a number of guided meditations that are available on YouTube absolutely free, and you can meditate in the comfort of your home. This is a wonderful way to get started practicing meditation without feeling uncomfortable. The YouTube meditations can help you if you don't really know how to mediate. But the best way to meditate is just to give yourself 20–30 minutes each day to focus on just relaxing by yourself without any stimulation of any kind. Start by relaxing your toenails and work your way up to your hair. The YouTube meditations that I enjoy help guide me through the process so I can concentrate on the process instead of trying to quiet my thoughts. Just remember to use your headphones so outside distractions are kept to a minimum.

- Walking—light exercise like walking helps to stimulate your digestive system. Have you been too sedentary? Take a walk to get your body and your bowels moving. Inactivity slows down the body processes. When you increase physical activity, you increase your breathing and heart rate. This in turn stimulates muscle contraction of your intestinal muscles, which will help you to go more easily and consistently, helping you to avoid constipation altogether.

- Read for enjoyment—pick a novel that is a guilty pleasure and relaxing. It will help to refocus your thoughts and get your mind in a more relaxed state. Do not pick a novel that has violence or too much negativity. You are trying to relax.

- Phone a friend that is fun and positive, not one that needs a lot of problem solving. A good positive conversation is uplifting and changes the focus of your day.

- Shopping at an *actual physical store* where you must walk around, look at what the store has to offer in person, and talk to actual people. Online shopping is terrific when you're in a time crunch and want easy and convenient shopping, but going to an actual store really does lift your mood, even if you are only window shopping or just trying on shoes or clothes for fun. We humans really do need interpersonal interaction with one another every day to stay mentally healthy. If shopping makes you stressed or grumpy visit a park and go for a long walk.

- Sign up and take a class at the community center. Try a dance class, yoga or maybe painting. A wonderful way to meet new friends, learn and relax.

- Coloring in a coloring book—when was the last time you colored? Coloring is such a great way to feel creative without the pressure of drawing or creating. It's one activity that just about anyone will enjoy and "get into" regardless of age or gender. It's great when the stress is on and you need to work something out or refocus. On one particular occasion, my husband and I took our daughter who was about 6 or 7 at the time, to a business meeting with us and brought a few coloring books, crayons, and colored pencils to have as activity for her during the meeting. She was always good in business meetings if we needed to take her along and was truly interested in what was being said.

Our clients watched her color while we discussed our business agendas and eventually, they couldn't resist anymore. One person asked our daughter if they could have a page out of her coloring book to color along with her. She happily tore out pages from her coloring book and customized what that person would like to color: boys got dragons, and I believe Pocahontas/Captain John Smith pages, and the girls got flowers and kitties. She gave them each a page to color along with an invitation to use her crayons and pencils.

We talked about business strategies and marketing as we all colored, and later everyone raved about their cool and relaxing meeting. The next time I went back for a meeting, the colored pages were displayed in the breakroom on the company refrigerator. So, don't underestimate the power of coloring, even for busy and important CEOs.

- Painting—you don't have to be an expert artist to experiment. Try watercolors or get a paint by numbers set if you need a little guidance to get started.
- Doing a puzzle—start off simple, and then work your way up to the complex pieces. You can find puzzles for a very reasonable price at garage sales & thrift stores.
- Playing a board game with friends—just make sure they aren't too cut-throat or competitive, as this can lead to more stress and tension. From what I understand, the game Monopoly is banned by the Queen of England in their household because things seemed to get a little too competitive, and

every time they played the game a not-so-royal conflict would break out among family members that was deemed "undignified for royal behavior."

- Put down your phone, especially before bedtime—don't look at social media while you are stressed. This is a time when the mind needs to calm down and not have additional stimulation. The blue light that the cell phone emits can actually disrupt your circadian rhythm and cause more stress in the long run. It also causes an addictive cycle because of the dopamine rush that "likes" can induce from social media approval. From what I understand, Dr. Oz does not allow cell phones in the bedroom because it is too disruptive to the sleep cycle.

I'm sure you see a little bit of a trend here. Engage in "real" activities, reduce your phone and computer time. Take time for you. Quiet your whole mind, body, and spirit for just a little while and *slow down*. It is important to nurture yourself to recharge your inner battery. For some this simple technique helps them to rejuvenate and feel less stressed, making the routine of pooping become pleasant and less stressful.

CHAPTER II: THE GUT BRAIN CONNECTION

You may have been hearing a lot about the gut-brain connection, as it has been a popular topic lately in news, magazines and social media.

Did you know? Anxiety and depression may contribute to conditions like IBS (irritable bowel syndrome)? If you have ever "gone with a gut feeling" in making a decision, or felt "butterflies in your stomach" when you were nervous or had anxiety, you may have been getting signals from the most unexpected source—your *second* brain. Where is this "second brain?" It is deep inside your digestive system and is revolutionizing understanding of the link between digestion, mood, health, and possibly even your thoughts.

Scientists are calling this brain in your gut the *enteric nervous system* (ENS). The ENS consists of two thin layers of more than 100 million nerve cells lining your gastrointestinal tract from esophagus to rectum.

What Does Your Gut's Brain Control?

The ENS has a different function than the brain in your head. It does not take on tasks like writing or computing numbers. The primary role is digestion, from the time food enters the mouth, through the release of enzymes that help break down food, all the way to elimination. Jay Pasricha, M.D., Director of the Johns Hopkins Center for Neurogastroenterology, whose research on the enteric nervous system has garnered international attention explains, "The enteric nervous system doesn't seem capable of thought as we know it, but it communicates back and forth with our big brain—with profound results."[8]

If you have irritable bowel syndrome (IBS) and experience problems like constipation, diarrhea, bloating, pain, and stomach upset, the ENS may trigger emotional shifts as well as gastrointestinal effects. "For decades, researchers and doctors thought that anxiety and depression contributed to these problems. But our studies and others show that it may also be the other way around," Pasricha says. [8] Research shows that irritation in the gastrointestinal system may send signals to the central nervous system (CNS) that trigger mood changes. "These new findings may explain why a higher-than-normal percentage of people with IBS and functional bowel problems develop depression and anxiety," Pasricha says. "That's important, because up to 30 to 40 percent of the population has functional bowel problems at some point." [1]

New Treatment Opportunities

ENS-CNS connection helps us to better understand IBS and treating bowel-disorder with antidepressants and mind-body therapies like cognitive behavioral therapy (CBT) and medical hypnotherapy. "Our two brains 'talk' to each other, so therapies that help one may help the other," Pasricha says. "In a way, gastroenterologists (doctors who specialize in digestive conditions) are like counselors looking for ways to soothe the second brain."

Gastroenterologists may prescribe antidepressants to help treat IBS, not because they think the patient has psychological issues, but because these antidepressants help to calm symptoms by acting on nerve cells in the gut, Pasricha explains. "Psychological interventions like CBT may also help to "improve communications" between the big brain and the brain in our gut," he says.

Physical Stresses You May Feel

- Stiff muscles in the neck and shoulders
- Headaches
- Sleep problems
- Feeling shaky or experiencing tremors
- Loss of interest in sex
- Weight loss or gain
- Feeling restless

Habits and Behaviors that You May Notice

- Putting off things, procrastination
- Grinding or gritting your teeth
- Having trouble completing work assignments
- Increase or decrease in alcohol or food you consume
- Starting to smoke or increasing smoking
- Wanting to be alone more
- Rumination—replaying stressful situations in life

The Emotions that You May Feel

- Feeling weepy
- Feeling pressured or too much tension
- Can't relax
- Feeling nervous
- Quick to anger or feeling irritated
- Feeling depression
- Lack of concentration
- Having trouble recalling things
- No sense of humor

- Can't make decisions—even easy ones

Stress can be a big factor in food digestion and pooping. Chronic stress and anxiety can take its toll even when digesting foods because of the gut-brain connection.

---

1. Hopkins Medicine. The brain-gut connection. Accessed July 16, 2020.

CHAPTER 12: DO POOPING HABITS CHANGE AS YOU AGE?

Many people, as they get older, start to experience trouble with constipation. This is due in part to a decrease in peristalsis, the contraction of the intestinal muscles, along with not enough fiber intake in the diet. Many people also do not drink enough water every day to keep their digestive tract hydrated and functioning properly.

Exercise is also a must as you get older, and it really does affect your ability to poop. Having good abdominal muscle tone is important in the overall health of your digestive system. It is common for the aging population to accept body changes like being a little heavier and less toned as you age. After all, you won't look like you did when you were 20. But the facts are, regardless of whether or not you put on a couple of pounds, it is important to exercise and to stay limber and firm—no matter your age. Just because your birthday cake is filled with so many candles it looks like you should call the fire department, it does not mean that you should let yourself go physically. Being too sedentary is not a good idea at any age. Stay as active and flexible as possible with simple strategies like a 30-minute walk and some light stretching. Yoga is another great way to keep flexibility and strength in focus. Keep your regime simple but consistent.

I remember an episode of Dr. Oz where he recommends that all ages be able to get off the floor without assistance, just using their legs to rise up. His advice is that if you keep your leg muscles strong, flexible, and limber, you will have less issues. It seems like a good idea for anyone that does not have knee or hip issues or cannot lift themselves safely by themselves.

With some people, lacking muscle tone in their core really affects the bowel muscle and can be the culprit of constipation problems. If this is the case, take a walk, do light weight-bearing exercises, eat fiber, and drink plenty of water to help stimulate muscle action to help with constipation.

Taking certain medications like blood pressure medications, antidepressants, pain medication, narcotics, antacids, and iron supplements can lead to constipation.

In our 'Supplements that Help Constipation' section there will be a few recommendations that have worked for me personally and for our family.

Please consult your physician before adding any supplements to your daily regime.

CHAPTER 13: DAILY POOP-PROMOTING TIPS

- Increase water intake to 8-10 glasses every day to hydrate the digestive system and you! Hydrating your digestive system is the key factor in helping constipation.

- Increase fiber intake—use age guidelines mentioned in the previous chapter. If you increase your fiber intake, remember you must drink water. Otherwise you will become more constipated.

- Include a cup of coffee or tea in the morning if you are able to drink caffeine. It helps stimulate bowels. If you can't drink coffee because of caffeine restrictions, just stick to water.

- Do not use flavored creamers I know, they are easy, convenient, don't go bad in the fridge, and they taste wonderful in your coffee. But they are filled with a bunch of not-good-for-you chemicals and additives. It really isn't "real food" in any sense. Just use half and half, cream, or a non-dairy almond, coconut, or cashew natural creamer. You could also try a flavored liquid stevia alternative like hazelnut or vanilla in your coffee or tea. I hear

Tim Tebow's favorite is vanilla liquid stevia in his coff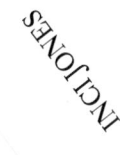 labels to make sure the natural creamer does not contain ~ of sugar.

- Sugar and sugar substitutes – The more you can reduce sug.   .r daily eating plan the better. Sugar helps to promote inflammauon and should be used in moderation and as sparingly as possible. It is unrealistic to say that you are going to have zero sugar in your diet, because if you eat a slice of bread, even if it's whole wheat, and homemade, the carbs convert to sugar in your body. If you have a piece of fruit, that converts to sugar in your body as well. But the goal in eating healthy is substituting the white sugar content that may be hidden in various foods for healthy alternatives. As always, read labels. If you are having coffee do not use the traditional flavored creamer. Use a flavored liquid stevia alternative like Hazelnut or Vanilla in your coffee or tea. I hear Tim Tebow's favorite is Vanilla liquid stevia in his coffee.

- Incorporate chicory coffee into your day. It helps to promote regularity and improve bowel function and reduce constipation. You can brew it with your coffee in the morning and it helps make your coffee taste smooth and less acidic. Or forego the coffee entirely and have it in lieu of anything caffeinated in the afternoon. Not only will it help with pooping, but you will be less stressed and have an easier time getting to sleep.

- Try a serving of vegetable soup for lunch, snack, or dinner. It's low-calorie, hydrating, delicious, filling, and you won't even realize you are eating your veggies.

- Include a serving of lentils or beans in your diet a few times a week. A perfect lunchtime meal, it fills you up and keeps you going, energy-wise. It's chock-full of fiber and protein that will keep you from snacking later in the afternoon. If you have trouble digesting beans, then give the digestive supplement Beano a try. It helps your body get used to digesting gas-inducing foods (fibery foods) and makes you less gassy.

• Have at least 1 serving of a green salad dressed with olive oil and balsamic vinegar (probiotics) or lemon juice. Add salt, pepper and garlic to your taste.

• No commercial dressings, because it may contain ingredients that "clog" your system like emulsifiers, flavor enhancers, or trans fats. The goal is to feed your body foods and beverages that replenish and pamper your body, not that further tax the digestive system.

• Indulge in eating hydrating foods like cucumbers, celery, lettuce, and zucchini when snacking instead of chips or bars.

• Add chickpeas or beans to salads and soups. They add great flavor and fill you up while giving you the additional fiber that helps keep you full. They help promote a healthy digestive system, producing an easy poop.

• Eat fruit for dessert—fruits like strawberries, grapes, watermelon, apricots, and oranges are helpful in keeping you unconstipated and going easily. Also include pineapple and papaya if they are in season. Both fruits are brimming with digestive enzymes and will help your digestive system get back on track to help you digest foods more efficiently. If you have any health concerns like diabetes and need to consider/account for fruit sugar intake, make sure to consult your physician with your dietetic questions and follow the serving sizes that are recommended by your physician or dietician.

• Try making your own bread if possible. Some of the commercially produced breads have wheat gluten, fillers, stabilizers, and dough conditioners that can cause a slowdown in your digestive system. Our family highly recommends the Zojirushi bread maker. Since we purchased our bread maker, I rarely purchase bread from the grocery store. It's so easy, I literally dump everything into the bread maker and it magically makes the most delicious breads, without chemicals. It literally takes 5 minutes to put all the ingredients into the bin. Less time than it takes to run to the market, stand in line at the checkout and purchase a loaf when you are out of bread. And the best part of making your own bread is the heavenly baking bread smell in your home. And with the prices of a loaf of bread these days, it really is quite economical as well.

Back in the early 2000's I had a bread maker, but the loaves were not really a usable shape (round) for sandwiches or just for toasting, so I really didn't use the old-style bread maker too much. The current bread maker that I use is the Zojirushi and it makes a beautiful loaf that is perfect for sandwiches and is wonderful for morning toast. This bread maker actually makes loaves, so it is not like the previous bread makers. I have included the bread maker in the Resource Section of this book for your convenience.

If you opt to purchase bread at the grocery store, please read the label—carefully. If you do not understand what the ingredients are, then don't buy it. You do not need those chemicals in your body. On occasion, when I actually purchase a loaf of bread from the grocery store, it's usually a sourdough bread without preservatives or Ezekiel bread. Our family likes the version with the sesame seeds. Ezekiel bread is not found in the bread section of the grocery store. It is usually stocked in the freezer section, because it does not contain chemicals and goes bad if you leave it out on the shelf. So, if you do purchase Ezekiel bread, store it in the refrigerator to keep it from spoiling. It's fabulous toasted with a smear of almond butter and a small dash of honey for a quick breakfast or snack.

Contrary to some commercially made loaves' claims that they are "all natural," they will actually stay fresh for months. Last Thanksgiving, time was of the essence, and I didn't have time to make homemade rolls. So, I purchased rolls for our meal that were labeled "natural." We ended up having some rolls left over after our dinner and left them in the bread drawer for over 3 months to see just how "natural" they were—and we were curious to see when the rolls would get moldy or go bad.

My daughter and I had a $5 bet, and both of us lost. The "natural" rolls never deteriorated or went bad. My daughter now refers to them as "Franken-Rolls" when we see them in the grocery store. Finally, I gave up on my experiment and threw them out because I was tired of seeing them there, and we both called it a draw and lost the bet. This in no way is a "natural" food. You should avoid eating this type of bread. Your body cannot process it as it is so indigestible that mold won't even grow on it. It is so synthetic that it does not deteriorate or decompose. Franken-Rolls!

CHAPTER 14: WHY YOU SHOULD BE DRINKING CHICORY COFFEE EVERY DAY

Chicory is a cousin of the dandelion family. Chicory coffee is made using chicory roots that are roasted, ground, and then brewed into a drink that tastes similar to coffee—minus the caffeine. Chicory contains small amounts B-6 and manganese, two nutrients that promote brain health. The root also contains inulin, a prebiotic fiber that helps not only to manage blood sugar levels, but also helps with digestion, constipation, and heart health.

History chronicles that France in the 1800's experienced massive coffee shortages. The ever-resourceful citizens of France, not one to skimp on flavor and the morning ritual, mixed chicory with their coffee to extend it, or substituted it for coffee entirely when none was available. Chicory can be used either on its own or mixed with coffee to complement and enhance its flavor, making it less acidic, and smoother in taste.

Marching forward to the Civil War in the United States, New Orleans residents began mixing coffee with chicory when the Union set up Naval blockades that cut off access to coffee shipments. When coffee supplies ran short, chicory made it a little less uncomfortable in the morning when coffee was hard to find. Chicory coffee is still popular around the world and a caffeine-free way to enjoy a coffee-like beverage.

I recently started drinking Chicory coffee in the afternoon to help with digestion and cut down on caffeine as even a cup of tea seemed to affect my evening sleep. After doing some research to see just how it benefits digestion and the pooping process, I learned that chicory could really help to improve bowel function and reduce constipation. The inulin in chicory helps to promote the growth of beneficial bacteria in the gut.

A recent study had 44 people with constipation supplement with chicory inulin. It was found to increase stool frequency and softness, compared to a placebo. In another study, consuming chicory decreased defecation difficulties among 25 elderly participants.[1]

From personal experience, I can report that chicory makes pooping easier, and the urge to poop is a natural feeling—not like the urgency you feel when taking a laxative.

Chicory coffee can be found on Amazon in instant, and you can also find the traditional ground root that you will need to steep like tea. Once the tea is brewed (5 minutes), then strain and drink like coffee, with creamer, stevia or with nothing at all. It has a natural sweetness that reminds me of maple syrup.

1. „„. Effect of consumption of chicory inulin on bowel function in healthy subjects with constipation: a randomized, double-blind, placebo-controlled trial. 2017 Feb; 68(1): 82–89. doi: 10.1080/09637486.2016.1212819. Epub 2016 Aug 5.

CHAPTER 15: HOW MUCH WATER DO YOU REALLY CONSUME?

We all know that we are supposed to drink water every day for good health. But are you really getting enough water for optimum digestive health? How can you tell if you are dehydrated? Most people are dehydrated and have no idea. The symptoms of subtle dehydration can be a slight headache or a little tiredness, and if you are more dehydrated, constipation. If you are dehydrated, it will cause constipation. I am repeating this, so it becomes second nature to you. If you are dehydrated, you will have constipation.

Drink water—not soda, not hydration drinks, and not fruit drinks. Drink water instead. Please keep track of how many glasses of water you are actually drinking in the beginning. You might be surprised to find out that you really aren't drinking enough water. If you are only drinking 3–4 glasses of water and think this is enough, that may be the reason you are constipated. And if you increase your fiber intake to help with constipation and don't drink enough water, you will become *more* constipated, because your body doesn't have enough water to move the poop out of the body. You essentially have just made a nice dry brick with the additional fiber, compounding the constipation that you are already experiencing. Your poop is just not hydrated because there is not enough water in the digestive tract.

A good start is 8–10 glasses of water per day to hydrate you and to ensure easier pooping. Some people may require a bit more water to get their intestines happy, hydrated, and pooping. If you are not good at drinking water, keep track for 30 days until it becomes second nature to you.

Another consideration…are you drinking excessive amounts of coffee, tea, energy drinks, or alcohol? These too can be a contributing factor in constipation. All of the above can be very dehydrating to your body. If you are having multiple cups of coffee and energy drinks during the day and 3–4 alcoholic drinks a night, you are dehydrated, and that may be the cause of your constipation. Some say with each cup of coffee or caffeinated beverage, you need to drink 2 glasses to compensate for the dehydration that it can cause.

Many times, the complaint is, "I hate drinking water because it does not taste like anything. It's so boring…I just can't drink it." If that is the case, flavor your water naturally. Make spa water for yourself. Add some cucumber slices, lemon, and mint. Let it set overnight for maximum flavor. Or another great way to add flavor is a few chunks of watermelon, strawberry, or orange slices. They all add great flavor.

You may also want to try a fruit juice spritzer. Add ¼ cup of juice to any natural sparkling water, add ice if you like, stir, and enjoy. It will hydrate you without a lot of sugar and maximum amount of taste.

CHAPTER 16: EAT A HYDRATING DIET

Another good way to hydrate your digestive system is by eating hydrating foods. There are a lot of fruits and vegetables, in a wide array of colors and flavors that contain not only water, but also provide many valuable nutrients, vitamins, minerals, and fiber that help to keep you healthy.

Here is a list of veggies & fruits and their water content [1]

Cucumbers—Water content: 96.73%

Cucumbers are a source of potassium, phosphorus, magnesium, and a small amount of calcium. They are not high in vitamin and mineral content compared to other veggies, but they do contain a special nutrient called cucurbitacin, which may have an anti-diabetic effect. Try adding cucumber to your water to add flavor.

Iceberg Lettuce—Water content: 95.64%

Even though this variety of lettuce is not as nutrient dense as some of its leafy green cousins, it still offers many benefits. It is low in carbs and sugar, contains fiber, vitamins A and K, potassium, and zinc. There are some that say that eating iceberg lettuce daily helps them fall asleep easier.

Celery —Water content: 95.43%

Celery is low in calories, protein, and carbohydrates and packed with loads of fiber. It is rich in vitamins A and K, folate and potassium. It's perfect for a cool, crunchy snack anytime. Celery is the perfect vehicle for peanut butter, almond butter, sunflower butter, or cream cheese.

Tomatoes—Water content: 94.52%

Is it a vegetable or a fruit? Even though I know it's a fruit, it seems to have more vegetable applications than a fruit in meals. Tomatoes are a fruit brimming with vitamins C and K, folate, and potassium. Tomatoes are also high in lycopene that helps prevent cell damage in the body. Tomatoes are one of the main sources of lycopene in the United States.

Romaine Lettuce—Water content: 93.47%

Romaine lettuce is a cousin to the iceberg lettuce variety and is just about neck and neck with iceberg in regard to water content. The darker leaves of romaine lettuce offers more nutritional benefits. It is a good source of vitamins A, C, and K, folate, and fiber.

Zucchini—Water content: 92.73%

Zucchini contains manganese, potassium, magnesium, Vitamin A, C, and K, and fiber.

It also contains antioxidants like lutein and zeaxanthin, which can help fight damage to the body's DNA.

Watermelon—Water content: 91.45%

Watermelon is THE summertime staple at any meal. Hydrating, sweet and just plain delicious. It's hydrating benefits are a great fit for hot weather.

No surprise to anyone, watermelon contains mostly water and some good for you vitamins like Vitamin A, C, several B vitamins, potassium, zinc, copper and a lot of other minerals.

Spinach—Water content: 91.4%

This small leafy green veggie has a whole host of nutrition and is low calorie too.

Spinach is a good source of magnesium, calcium, iron, potassium, vitamins A and K, fiber, and folate. Perfect for salads, smoothies, cooked in quiches, omelets and sauces.

Strawberries—Water content: 90.95%

Sweet, fragrant, and delicious strawberries, chock-full of fiber, vitamin C, and antioxidants that help your body fight damage from free radicals.

Skim Milk—Water content: 90.84%

Skim milk is a healthy beverage to drink in cereals or as a pick-me-up snack for a quick shot of protein. Skim milk is a good way to contribute to your calcium and vitamin D intake for the day.

Soy Milk—Water content: 90.36%

Soy milk is a mixture of water and soybeans that makes for a milk substitute beverage.

Soy milk from the grocery store is usually fortified with added calcium, vitamin D, and several B vitamins.

Cantaloupe—Water content: 90.15%

Cantaloupe is the perfect summertime or anytime addition to meals or snacks. It is high in vitamin C and a good source of beta carotene, which the body converts to vitamin A.

Honeydew Melon—Water content: 89.82%

This sweet, green melon with a slight cucumber taste is high in potassium, vitamins C and K, folate, and magnesium.

Kale—Water content: 89.63%

If you've visited a grocery store lately, I'm sure you've noticed that kale has taken front and center stage in the vegetable department. You can find it ready to use, chopped and bagged. Just pop it into a salad bowl, toss, and eat. Simple! Here's the reason why kale is so popular—it is a nutrient-dense, leafy green vegetable, high in vitamins A, B, C, and K. It is also a good source of calcium, fiber, protein, iron, anti-inflammatory phytochemicals, and omega-3 fatty acids. Kale is a wonderful source of iron, vitamin B and anti-inflammatory phytochemicals.

Broccoli—Water content: 89.3%

Broccoli is definitely not at the top of many people's list of favorite foods to eat, but did you know broccoli contains almost 90% water! It also contains many different antioxidants, fiber, iron, potassium, and vitamins C and K.

Peaches—Water content: 88.87%

When peach season rolls around, our family is truly excited. Nothing is better than a tree-ripened peach! This delicious fruit contains a whole array of vitamins A, C, E, and K and is a good source of potassium and phosphorus. It's easy to eat on the go or incorporate into shakes, salads, salsa, or chutney.

Carrots—Water content: 88.29%

Carrots are delicious eaten raw and crunchy, slathered with hummus or yogurt dip. Or you can cook them in stir-fry's or desserts. Grate into spaghetti sauce to add flavor, fiber, and vitamins. Even carrot dislikers won't detect they're in the sauce. Carrots are high in vitamins A and K, folate, potassium, and fiber. And they are definitely not only for rabbits.

Oranges—Water content: 86.75%

During the winter, how many times have you been reminded to drink your orange juice to help keep the cold or flu at bay? A better alternative would be to eat an actual orange. Not only will you get your vitamin C to help prevent colds and flu, but you will also get the wonderful fiber that each orange contains. Oranges are also rich in potassium, vitamin B, magnesium, selenium, and copper. Plus, peeling an orange gives a whole different meaning to aromatherapy. Just breathe in the heavenly smell as you peel.

Pineapple—Water content: 86%

When you want a special touch to any meal or snack, splurge on a whole pineapple.

Although pineapple can look a bit intimidating to peel, it's well worth the effort. Pineapple is packed with vitamin C, magnesium, potassium, manganese, and vitamin B. It also contains an enzyme called bromelain that has wonderful anti-inflammatory effects.

Many people that want to improve their digestion include pineapple in their diet.

Apples—Water content: 85.56%

Every fall when apple season arrives, it is your chance to enjoy all of the varieties of apples—from green, pink, red, to ruby red. Each has an individual flavor and crunch. Apples are a wonderful source of water, contain fiber, vitamin C, and antioxidants like quercetin and catechin.

---

1. Medical News Today. Hydrating foods: the top 20 and their benefits. undefinedundefined Accessed July 16, 2020.

CHAPTER 17: ARE PRESCRIPTION DRUGS OR OTC'S CAUSING YOUR CONSTIPATION?

Some of the most common OTC (over the counter) drugs can cause constipation.

- Did you know that pain relievers or NSAIDs (non-steroidal anti-inflammatory drugs) like ibuprofen and aspirin may cause constipation?
- A little indigestion? Antacid tablets to soothe your acidy stomach, especially calcium and aluminum-containing antacids, can contribute to constipation.
- Speaking of acidy stomach, if you take an acid reducer to help relieve acid reflux or an acidy stomach, it can be another contributor to constipation. A relative of ours has problems with acid reflux and takes a couple of Tums for immediate relief, then a Pepcid to help relieve the acid feeling in

the stomach and throat for the rest of the day. This combination can lead to constipation.

• Allergy season...and you take an antihistamine like Benedryl, Claritin, Zyrtec etc? Antihistamines like diphenhydramine and the like can cause constipation.

• Do your nutritional supplements contain iron? If yes, then that may contribute to constipation.

Prescription Drugs that May Contribute to Constipation

• Opioid pain-relievers, like morphine, codeine etc.

• Anti-cholinergic agents like atropine, trihexyphenidyl

• Antispasmodics, like dicyclomine

• Tricyclic antidepressants, like amitriptyline

• Calcium channel blockers used in arrhythmias and high blood pressure such as verapamil

• Anti-Parkinsonian drugs—Parkinson's disease itself may cause constipation, and the drugs used for this condition, including levodopa, cause constipation as well.

• Sympathomimetics, like ephedrine and terbutaline. Terbutaline is commonly used on bronchial asthma.

• Antipsychotics, like clozapine, thioridazine, chlorpromazine used for psychiatric disorders

• Diuretics for heart failure, like furosemide

• High blood pressure lowering agents, like methyldopa, clonidine, propranolol etc.

• Antidiarrheal agents, like loperamide and attapulgite

• Anticonvulsants, like phenytoin and clonazepam

• Miscellaneous compounds including octreotide, polystyrene resins, cholestyramine (for lowering high blood cholesterol), and oral contraceptives

If you are taking any of the prescription medication in the above list you may need to not only to implement the changes in diet and water intake, relaxation techniques that are suggested, but also the products that I used when I was on chemotherapy. As I mention later, the constipation from the anti-nausea, pain and other medications really made me constipated.

CHAPTER 18: IS YOUR CALCIUM SUPPLEMENT CAUSING CONSTIPATION?

Below is a calcium cheat sheet from Arthritis.org that is helpful in defining calcium intake and type of calcium that is most beneficial for bone maintenance and least constipating.

Calcium Supplement Basics

If your doctor recommends you take a calcium supplement, here are some tips to know before you buy:

1. Understand how much calcium you are getting through your diet before you take supplements. Taking too much can be bad for you.

2. Take several smaller doses per day, because your body can absorb only 500 mg at a time.

3. Your body needs vitamin D to use calcium most efficiently, so look for supplements that contain both.

Calcium "Cheat Sheet" There are several different types of calcium. Check out the chart below for the three most popular types, and to help determine the best calcium supplement for you. Other kinds, such as calcium gluconate and calcium lactate, have very low amounts of elemental calcium and are not recommended. Coral calcium and oyster-shell calcium products also are best avoided because they may contain lead.

Calcium Guide

Calcium Type	Pros	Cons
Calcium Citrate 21% Calcium Like Citrical, Solgar	Most easily absorbed	Most Expensive, doesn't contain much elemental calcium
Calcium Citrate 21% Calcium Like Tums, Caltrate, Rolaids	Least Expensive, has more elemental calcium	Take with meals or glass of acidic orange juice, may cause gas or constipation
Calcium phosphate 39% Calcium Like Posture	Does not cause gas or constipation, easily absorbed	More expensive than calcium carbonate

Precautions: Don't take more than 1,200 mg of calcium (in supplement form) a day unless instructed by a doctor or dietitian. Also, avoid taking calcium supplements at the same time as some kinds of medications, including bisphosphonates, like alendronate (*Fosamax*) and ibandronate (*Boniva*) and certain antibiotics, because it can block their absorption by the body. As with any supplement, talk to your doctor before taking. [1]

---

1. Arthritis Foundation. Calcium needs for people with arthritis. https://www.arthritis.org/about-arthritis/types/osteoporosis/articles/calcium-supplements.php . Accessed January 27, 2020.

CHAPTER 19: YOU'VE BEEN HEARING ABOUT IT...LEAKY GUT. WHAT IS IT?

The intestinal lining covers more than 4,000 square feet of surface area in our digestive tract and when working properly makes a tight barrier that controls what gets absorbed into our bloodstream. Leaky gut syndrome or "intestinal permeability," describes the condition of the intestinal lining becoming more porous. If gut lining is unhealthy it may have large cracks, holes, or fissures that allow partially digested food and toxins to penetrate the tissues. When you have a leaky gut condition, the damaged microvilli along the intestinal lining cannot manufacture the digestive enzymes they need to break down the food for proper digestion. This could trigger an inflammation response and change the normal gut flora and bacteria that could lead to trouble in the digestive system and other areas of the body. [1]

Who Is Susceptible to Leaky Gut?

Many people may have a mild form of leaky gut and only notice occasionally that something doesn't feel right or comfortable. Most of us might dismiss this as, "I just ate something that didn't agree with me." But a certain segment of the population may have a genetic predisposition to leaky gut and have a digestive system that is more sensitive to any minor change.

Our modern diet may actually help to promote gut inflammation. So, genetics may not be the only cause. The American diet is usually low in fiber, high in sugar, full of saturated fats, and laced with chemicals and ingredients that may help to instigate the leaky gut process. Stress, drinking caffeine and alcohol also help add to the mix.

It is common knowledge that increased intestinal permeability plays a role in certain gastrointestinal conditions such as celiac disease, Crohn's disease, and irritable bowel syndrome. The question is whether or not leaky gut can cause problems elsewhere in the body. Recent studies show that leaky gut may be associated with other autoimmune diseases, such as lupus, type 1 diabetes, multiple sclerosis, chronic fatigue syndrome, fibromyalgia, arthritis, allergies, asthma, acne, obesity, and mental illness.

Promoting A Healthier Gut

An initial step most practitioners implement is elimination of foods that can cause inflammation and may promote undesirable gut flora changes. Among the most common to eliminate are caffeine, alcohol, processed foods that contain chemicals and additives, some medications, and any foods that may cause the body allergies or sensitivities like dairy, eggs, and wheat. There is some controversy whether leaky gut causes the development or progression of diseases outside of the gastrointestinal tract in humans. The key is eating a fresh and nutritious diet of unprocessed foods that help reduce inflammation. Keep your diet as simple and natural as possible, include a variety of vegetables, and avoid foods that may trigger inflammation by being aware of foods as you eat them. Do you experience discomfort after eating? That is a tell-tale sign that this food may not be agreeing with your body. Avoid "trigger foods" that further irritate the digestive system and cause digestive issues and constipation or diarrhea. Being mindful of your diet can help to rebuild the gut lining and bring balance to the gut flora.

What Foods to Avoid if You Have Leaky Gut

Eating foods that reduce inflammation help heal your gut. Trigger foods can cause symptoms to progress and become worse over time if consumption continues. After repeated exposure to the trigger foods, the body then develops the inflammatory response to protect itself. A lifetime of consuming the trigger foods can then lead to intestinal damage. But the good news is, the body can heal most minor damage if you are willing to make a few changes to your diet.

If you have leaky gut syndrome, below are seven foods that you should avoid or delete from your diet entirely.[2] This will help the body heal from the inflammation response and start to repair your intestinal tract, leaving it working optimally.

1. Sugar

This isn't the first time that you've heard that sugar may not be such a good idea in your diet, and you should cut down or avoid it altogether. But eating sugar with leaky gut promotes candida yeast production in the body, which in turn can cause fungal infections.

Candida overgrowth is fed by sugar and having a diet that is high in sugar can promote candida growth and worsen leaky gut syndrome. Also, do not use artificial sweeteners. You may want to sweeten with stevia, as it promotes gut health. Artificial sweeteners can promote an inflammatory reaction in the body or start a cavalcade of allergic responses in many people. Raw fruit or unpasteurized honey may also be used. But try small amounts to see if you can tolerate them.

2. Processed Oils

Include cold-pressed oils like olive oil and sesame oil in your anti-inflammatory leaky gut diet. Avoid highly processed soybean oil, corn oil, vegetable oil, and peanut oil. The high heating process during manufacturing kills nutrients and health benefits that are in the fat.

Other fats, like partially hydrogenated vegetable oils, margarine, and shortening are not permitted. These fats are not nutritionally valuable and promote gut inflammation.

3. Legumes

Many people have a sensitivity to beans, lentils, soybeans, and peanuts due to their high fiber content, making it a little difficult for the body to digest. I'm sure that we all have experienced gas after eating beans. So, if your gut is already weakened, not only will it cause excessive gas, but these foods can also inhibit healing. It may be best to avoid eating this food group to help promote healing at first. Then add them back in at a later time when your gut is healed and ready to take on the fiber of legumes.

4. Grains

We've all seen gluten-free foods on the grocery shelf and in restaurants, and we've heard how many people can have an intolerance to gluten. Even if you do not have celiac disease, you may still have an intolerance to gluten. Grains and flours like wheat, whole grain, and white flour contain gluten, and you should avoid products made with these flours.

When you are in the initial stages of healing a leaky gut, it is best to avoid all grains. You can re-introduce grains at a later time, if you would like to re-incorporate them into your diet.

5. Dairy

Many people have some degree of lactose intolerance but aren't aware of it. If you experience gas, flatulence, nausea, diarrhea, and constipation after you consume dairy products, that may be an indicator that you have lactose intolerance. The inflammatory response can occur when you consume milk, cream, butter, cheese, or any other product that contains a dairy source.

Replace these dairy products with non-dairy alternatives to make the transition easier on your taste buds and to help heal the gut and promote gut health. If you take milk or half and half in your coffee, try an almond milk alternative. Stay away from non-dairy, flavored creamers that have ingredients full of chemicals that are not natural. Remember, the key to healing is staying as natural as possible. Meaning...if you don't understand what the ingredients are on the back of the package...don't buy it, and definitely don't consume it!

6. Nightshade Vegetables

When you hear the word nightshade, Morticia from the Adams Family comes to mind with her rather unconventional garden. But in reality, vegetables in the nightshade family include everyday veggies that we all eat like potatoes, tomatoes, eggplant, peppers, and black pepper that you use to season your food. But not all vegetables in the nightshade family can cause problems. Because everyone is different in their sensitivity levels of these vegetables, you will need to do a trial to see if your trigger is potatoes or tomatoes. For my neighbor it was a common seasoning—black pepper.

Some vegetables in this family may not affect you, and you may be able to include them in your everyday diet. The nightshade family of vegetables are actually related to plants like belladonna. Nightshades contain an alkaloid called solanine, which is toxic in high concentrations. Solanine is found in trace amounts in potatoes and is normally safe. A 2010 study suggests that eating purple or yellow potatoes may reduce inflammation.[13] They contain high levels of antioxidants including carotenoids, which may help to prevent cell damage.

Some great substitutes when you eliminate nightshades from your diet are:

- sweet potatoes
- yams
- cauliflower

- mushrooms

7. Corn

Eating corn on the cob is *not* a no-no. But, corn with butter slathered all over the golden kernels (so delicious) is! But not really the most nutritious vegetable in the veggie world, and for some it can be hard to digest because it is fibrous and a little irritating to the digestive tract, if it is already irritated.

The main issue with corn is that it can be highly processed, like in corn meal. Corn, like soy, is found in many processed foods from breakfast cereals to chips and even frozen dinners. Because corn is inserted into so many processed foods as a thickener or filler, it is easy to develop an allergy or intolerance to corn. The best remedy for this is to avoid processed foods, especially those made with corn and soy. This elimination is necessary to protect your gut health and start the road to healing and well-being.

Trigger Foods?

Everyone's tolerance to trigger foods is individual. If you have leaky gut syndrome, you will need to identify your specific triggers by an elimination diet and slowly reintroduce foods on the above list to see what specific triggers are. This will give you a barometer on what is okay for you and what the trigger foods are that start the inflammation process in your body. The ultimate goal is to keep your body in a state of balance as much as possible to maintain gut health and healing at all times.

Foods to Eat Instead

Some of the best diets for gut health include the paleo diet or keto diet. These diets consist of a basic diet that includes meat, cheese, vegetables, and nuts. They do not include low-fat dairy, grains, legumes, sweets, or processed foods. Check out paleo or keto diet recipe books online to help you transition into the keto/paleo lifestyle.

I do have to make a side comment here about the excess fat consumption in both of these diets. Individuals that have used these particular diets have shared that they had to tone down the amount of fat that is sometimes suggested, because it caused some discomfort in their digestive system. So, tailor these plans to your comfort level and what works for you individually. Within the paleo lifestyle, there are foods that are nurturing to gut health and helping to reverse leaky gut syndrome:

1. Bone Broth

I'm sure you've seen and heard about the big trend on drinking bone broth. It seems that everyone is drinking this delicious elixir of health and healing. But I'm here to tell you...get on the bandwagon too! It's not just a fad—bone broth *is* actually good for you.

Bone broth can be nurturing to the intestinal tract, and it can improve gut health. It is made by slow cooking an assortment of bones in salted water that contains vegetables, eggshells, apple cider vinegar, and sea salt for many hours.

Did you know that bone broth is not only very tasty to sip but it is also brimming with nutrients? When bones are slow cooked for an extended period of time, they naturally release gelatin, calcium, glutamine, collagen, and a whole host of good for you nutrients. This lovely combo helps to replenish and rebuild the gut lining. The gelatin that occurs in bone broth is a hydrophilic colloid that holds liquids, which includes digestive juices. It also contains chondroitin sulfates, glucosamine, and other compounds that are extracted from the long cooking times when simmering the bones and cartilage.

Bone broth is packed with amino acids such as glycine, proline, and arginine, which all have anti-inflammatory properties that help the body heal. And if you are trying to boost your calcium and magnesium intake, bone broth can help with this as well.

Bone broth is simple and easy to make. The best way to make the broth is from organic, grass-fed beef and chicken bones. It is the perfect afternoon beverage to sip instead of coffee, tea, or an energy drink, and can be used as the base in a soup for lunch or dinner.

2. Steamed Vegetables

Eat your vegetables...bet you have heard that before. But vegetables are *vital* to your good health. They not only provide you with vitamins and minerals, but provide your gut the fiber to keep you regular and brush your system clean. Include a variety of multi-colored vegetables in your diet.

If you are not used to eating them, start with vegetables that are more on the bland side, like cooked green beans, salads, and cucumbers. Then work up to ones that have a more distinct taste like broccoli or cabbage. As you are finding out, they are an essential and nutritious part of gut recovery and healthy eating.

The best cooking method is steaming your vegetables till they are crisp but tender. This allows vegetables to retain their optimal nutritional value while making them easier to digest. Try tossing your veggies once they are steamed in a little olive oil or grass-fed cow butter, sea salt, and garlic. With all that flavor meshing and combining with your veggies, you'll feel like you are at a five-star restaurant. Ultimately vegetables contain essential nutrients that help the gut to heal, cruciferous vegetables like broccoli and cabbage, can aid in gut health and regeneration.

3. Probiotic Foods

The most important part of maintaining gut health is promoting good intestinal bacteria and decreasing the undesirable bacteria. Replacing the bad bacteria with good bacteria in the gut. The natural way to accomplish this is by including probiotics in your diet.

Probiotics are the beneficial bacteria that help your gut to protect and maintain its health. There are many probiotic supplements that you can include in your diet and are available at most stores.

But another way to promote good bacteria is eating fermented foods. Most people are familiar with the fact that yogurt contains probiotics, but if you have an intolerance to dairy, there are other options like almond or coconut milk yogurt yogurt. Coconut milk kefir is also a wonderful alternative to yogurt.

There are other fermented foods that are great for gut health like kimchi, sauerkraut, or fermented pickles.

4. Coconut Oil

Coconut oil is great at controlling and killing off candida overgrowth and one of the best foods for gut healing. Coconuts contain lauric acid, which contains antimicrobial and antifungal properties. Use coconut oil as a good alternative to butter and other cooking oils, as its anti-inflammatory properties help to soothe the intestine and reduce autoimmune response throughout the body.

5. Fish Oil

Fish oil is another component in rebooting and repairing your gut health. It is important to include healthy fats like fish oil into your diet. Try to include fish that you actually eat into your diet, and don't solely rely on fish oil supplements. One of the best sources of omega-3s are herring and anchovies, as they help reduce inflammation and improve gut health. Other types of fish that are rich in omega-3 fatty acids are salmon, tuna, trout, and mackerel. If you *do* opt to include fish oil supplements, please read the label to make sure that they are mercury-free fish oils.

6. Grass-Fed Meats

When possible, choose grass-fed and free-range meats and avoid beef and chicken that have been fed corn and soy products in their feed. Purchasing meat that has been carefully raised may be a bit more expensive, but your meats will be superior in quality with flavor that the corn-fed version does not have. Grass-fed meat also will have more CLA (conjugated linoleic acid), which is important for body metabolism and digestion. The most important reason to switch to grass-fed and free-range meats is to encourage your gut to return to comfort and health.

7. Processed and Cured Meats

Avoid cured processed meats and deli lunch meat at all costs. Most tradition-al bacon, ham, lunch meats, hot dogs, and sausage that you find in the grocery store contain nitrates. Read the labels carefully. There are a wide variety of natural brands that do not contain nitrates.

After doing a bit of research and trying out a few brands, our family really enjoys the Boar's Head brand of deli meats. Our local grocery store carries the whole line of Boar's Head deli meats. In my research I contacted the Boar's Head company directly to find out if any of their meats contain nitrates, and the only deli meat that does is their turkey ham. But the rest of their deli meat line does not.

Many grocery stores carry Boar's Head. Definitely add a natural brand to your grocery shopping list. The natural brands taste better, fresher, cleaner, and more like food and less like a chemical taste. You won't notice that you changed brands when you eat, but your body will thank you for not including the chemicals and additives.

1.
2.

CHAPTER 20: REMEMBER TO BE MINDFUL

Be mindful of the foods you are eating at all meals and snacks. Remember you are eating to live...not living to eat. During the time of rebuilding gut health, make sure that every bite is filled with natural nutrition that promotes nurturing and healing.

Make meals simple with the basics of a meat serving and a couple of different vegetables—all simple and easy to prepare. Try slow cooking the meat and vegetables if you don't have time to cook because of work or other commitments. Many people opt for the InstaPot or a traditional stovetop pressure cooker to speed up the cooking process. When you use an InstaPot or a pressure cooker, more vitamins are retained in the foods that you eat. It makes for fast, flavorful meals like stews and soups, and even meatloaf becomes effortless and quick to make.

Remember, good health is not overnight, but a step by step process. A wise saying that I love comes to mind from Earl Nightingale, "Time will pass anyway." With each day make your body healthier and an efficient running machine, instead of promoting wear, tear and unhealthy habits." In a few short weeks you will start to feel better, and in a few months, you will start to feel more energetic and see a big difference in the way your body processes the foods that you eat *and* how you poop.

CHAPTER 21: EXAMPLE MEAL PLAN

Easy Eating Plan for the Day:

The below menu is an example meal, you can adjust to your schedule.

Upon Arising:

1 glass of warm water with 1 tsp lemon juice—drink the whole glass before having breakfast.

Breakfast:

Coffee or tea—sweetened with stevia. You may add a dash of heavy cream or all-natural creamer like almond or coconut milk or half and half.

1-2 eggs—Prepare however you prefer, using olive oil or grass-fed cow butter.

1 slice of bread—Homemade, Ezekiel Bread, or natural Sourdough bread

1 serving (1/2 cup) fruit—Watermelon, strawberry or blueberry.

Lunch

1 bowl of homemade vegetable soup—Minestrone is a favorite in our home. We also make broccoli cheddar soup, which is another favorite. Make a quick soup in your slow cooker, pressure cooker, or InstaPot and have a ready-made soup for a few days for a fast and easy lunch at home or in the office. All you have to do is heat and eat.

(optional) Protein serving of 3-4 ounces—about the size of a deck of cards. This can be chicken, turkey, or fish. It is optional if you don't really feel like eating the protein at lunch.

Avocado Toast—1 slice of one of the bread selections above with ¼–½ avocado smushed on the bread. Season your avocado toast with sea salt and pepper, and a little drizzle of olive oil if you would like.

Handful of organic grapes or an apple for dessert

Snack

Orgain protein—Shake any flavor (we like vanilla), add kale, pineapple, blueberries, and strawberries. If you can't add the fruit, just the shake mix is great for an afternoon protein pick-me-up to keep from snacking and provide pea protein fiber to help with digestion. One of the Orgain Protein shake mixes contains a probiotic that is fabulous to keep the digestive system happy while your energy stays high and blood sugar remains balanced for the afternoon.

Dinner

Chicken, lamb, or fish broiled or lightly pan sautéed—lightly seasoned with herbs, sea salt, and pepper—Try to purchase chicken and lamb that is raised as organically as possible, and with the fish do not purchase farm-raised fish as they may contain antibiotics and can be high in PCB's and pesticides. In some countries that produce farm-raised fish they may be raised in unhygienic, contaminated water that is unhealthy.

Vegetable side dish like green beans, asparagus, zucchini squash, and mushrooms, stir-fried in a little olive oil or steamed—ry to purchase organic, non-GMO vegetables and ingredients.

Dinner salad—your choice of greens of any kind (organic is preferable), like romaine, baby kale, spinach with tomatoes, cucumbers, grated carrots and beets. You can add any vegetables into your salad that you enjoy eating. Try and focus on vegetables that have fiber and a high-water content. You can dress it with HHD (healthy house dressing) or our other favorite, poppyseed dressing. See next chapter for recipes.

CHAPTER 22: THE RECIPES

When you put your health and wellness above everything, you realize one thing. It's really not that hard to eat healthy, and the food that you eat is truly delicious and satisfying to your body, mind, and soul.

A good friend of ours made a comment to my husband the other day that was brilliant. My husband and Diane were discussing some of the restaurants in our area, and the fact that the food just didn't seem very healthy or delicious. Diane had some friends from out of town over, and of course they were eager to try some of the local restaurants. Diane, being health conscious, said, "Oh we'd love to go out, but Al (her husband) is on a restricted diet for his health, so it's too hard for him to eat out these days." This gave her and Al the perfect out for not eating at a restaurant, and people didn't feel uncomfortable about it. After all, everyone assumed that her husband couldn't eat out due to a doctor's recommendation. But really, the only health condition Diane had in mind was good, healthy eating, and she wanted to control the meal choice. This was a graceful and brilliant way to control eating options to accommodate health and wellness goals while not being impolite.

Below are some recipes that our family enjoys, and they are healthy, tasty, and easy to prepare.

Healthy House Dressing (HHD)

¼ cup rice vinegar

1 cup cold-pressed sesame oil

1-2 cloves chopped garlic

½ tsp grated fresh ginger

1-2 dashes soy sauce

Sea salt and fresh ground pepper to taste

Instructions

Combine all ingredients in a jar, close lid and shake. Store in refrigerator.

Another recipe that is in our fridge at all times is THE Poppyseed Dressing. It is a little old school, because it requires that you combine almost all of the ingredients and cook them for about 5 minutes in a saucepan. But it is totally worth the slightly extra effort because it tastes delicious! It's the perfect dressing for kale salads, because it tenderizes the kale if you leave it in the fridge overnight. It's perfect for next day lunches or dinner.

THE Poppyseed Dressing

2/3 cup water

¼ cup apple cider vinegar—like Braggs Apple Cider Vinegar

1 tsp of stevia

1 tsp olive oil

½ tsp sea salt

2 tsp corn starch

¼ tsp onion powder

½ tsp mustard powder

¼ tsp poppy seeds

1 Tbsp Hollywood Mayonnaise—I only use this mayo because it tastes so good!

Instructions

In a saucepan combine water, apple cider vinegar, stevia, olive oil, salt, corn starch, onion powder, and mustard powder on low heat until thickened. Add the poppy seeds. Whisk. Add the Hollywood mayo and whisk again till smooth. Decant into a jar and cool on the countertop. Keep in the refrigerator until use.

I love to use this dressing on kale salads, as it tenderizes the kale and gives it a great flavor. In fact, if you make the kale salad a day ahead of use, it is full of flavor and extra tender the next day. You will need to make it ahead of time if you plan on using it on lettuce, as it will need to cool in the fridge before using. It's not hard, I promise...and it's really worth the extra step.

If you want a truly filling and satisfying soup, then this is the recipe for you. This evolved one day when it was cold and blustery outside, and the snow just didn't seem like it would ever stop. I thought a soup would be the perfect warming thing to have for a family lunch since we were stuck inside.

I scoured the Internet to see what was available, and I came upon a few recipes that I liked. Over the last year or so I have honed the recipe and made a few adjustments to customize to our preferences to include a few more veggies than most recipes. Here is my version below.

Minestrone Soup

2 medium carrots, chopped

2 large stalks of celery, chopped

1 cup roughly chopped cauliflower

1 tsp of garlic, chopped

1 medium onion, diced

1-2 tsp dried basil

1 tsp dried oregano

1/2 tsp dried rosemary

1 tsp dried thyme

1 32-oz can fire roasted diced tomatoes

2 Tbsp tomato paste

3 bay leaves

32-oz carton (4 cups) low sodium vegetable broth

1-2 cups water—as needed to cover all the veggies

sea salt and freshly ground black pepper to taste

2 zucchini squash, quartered

1 can red kidney beans, rinsed and drained

1 can cannellini beans or great northern beans, rinsed and drained

1 can green beans

1-2 c fresh baby spinach, chopped

1 tsp balsamic vinegar (optional but adds great flavor)

shredded or grated Parmesan cheese for serving

fresh parsley, finely chopped, for garnish (optional)

Instructions

SLOW COOKER:

1. In a large 6-quart slow cooker, add the veggies - carrots, celery, onions, chopped garlic basil, oregano, rosemary, thyme, bay leaves, tomato paste and diced tomatoes. Pour the vegetable broth and water into the slow cooker and season with salt and pepper. Cover with a lid and cook on HIGH for 2-3 hours or LOW for 5-6 hours.

2. 20-30 minutes before serving, stir in kidney beans, cannellini beans, green beans, and zucchini, and continue cooking for an hour or two.

3. Stir in spinach at this point and taste to see if you need to season with more salt and pepper. Stir in balsamic vinegar last, and serve. You can top the soup with parmesan cheese to really add flavor.

This version works really well on the stove top. Nothing like a pot of soup simmering on the stove. Just add the ingredients in the same order. Cook for 20 minutes, and then add the other veggies and beans to cook for another 10 minutes, and *voila*—your soup is done.

Another favorite soup in our rotation is the broccoli cheddar soup that is similar to Panera's—only healthier and tastier. Even if you have a broccoli hater, this soup will change their minds with the first bite. We hope you'll love it as much as we do.

Just as a note—broccoli is NOT my husband's favorite vegetable, but he actually *asks me* to make this soup. Just letting you know.

Broccoli Cheddar Soup

2 cups low-sodium vegetable stock or chicken stock

4 c broccoli florets, chopped into smaller bite-sized pieces1 medium yellow onion, diced 1 tsp garlic, chopped

2 large carrots, sliced into rounds

salt to taste½ tsp freshly ground black pepper 1 tsp smoked paprika or regular paprika 1 ½ tsp dry mustard powder

1/2 c all-purpose flour1 c organic half and half

1 Tbsp grass-fed butter1 c grated organic extra-sharp cheddar cheese

Instructions:

1. In a large, heavy-bottom pot, add the vegetable or chicken stock. Add the broccoli, onions, garlic, and carrots. Add salt, pepper, paprika and dry mustard. Stir to incorporate all seasonings into soup mixture. Simmer for 10 minutes.

2. In another bowl, combine flour and half and half. Whisk thoroughly to eliminate lumps.

3. Add the flour and milk mixture to the soup—stirring constantly until incorporated. Add butter.Then simmer over low heat for about 20 to 25 minutes, stirring frequently or until it has reduced and thickened.

4. After soup simmers, add the grated cheese and stir. Reserve some cheddar cheese for topping the soup bowls later.

The soup will keep up to 7 days in the fridge. I haven't tried freezing the soup because A) We eat it too fast! and B) it contains half and half and I have not had good experiences with freezing meals made with cheese and half and half (it usually curdles as it thaws.) So just a warning for those who like to freeze their meals for meal prepping. If you have success with freezing creamy soups, please let me know your secret!

Buckwheat Grain Bread—Bread Machine Recipe

Makes a 2-pound loaf

1 ½ c very warm water from tap, not boiling

2 Tbsp butter, softened

1 ½ c all-purpose white flour

1 ½ c whole wheat flour

½ c buckwheat cereal (uncooked)

1 Tbsp molasses

1 ½ tsp salt

2 ½ tsp bread machine yeast

Instructions:

Place all ingredients in the bread machine in the order recommended by your manufacturer. Select "Wheat" setting or "White" setting with medium crust. Depending upon your climate, you may need more wheat flour or a little less. Cool on a rack for at least 15 minutes when finished cooking.

CHAPTER 23: WHEN THE GOING GETS TOUGH

If you are currently constipated, here are some tips to help you.

- Drink 8-10 glasses of water per day to hydrate your body and digestive system.
- Reduce refined carbohydrates like pre-packaged snacks and foods. Read labels to see if they contain ingredients that are 'real'. Anything with white flour, casein or other ingredients that you can't pronounce should be avoided.
- Eat foods that hydrate your body like watermelon, grapes, cucumbers, lettuce, apples, plums and apricots.
- Be sure to include fiber in your diet like beans and legumes.
- Incorporate one soup meal into your daily diet.
- Take a glucomannan supplement. If you're constipated, try taking a glucomannan supplement or eating shirataki noodles, which are made with

glucomannan. They look just like noodles and are wonderful alternatives in a ramen or spaghetti type dish.

• Include Prebiotic foods into your daily regime, like bananas, onions, and garlic.

• Eat 3 prunes every day. Not only will you enjoy the poop-promoting wonderfulness of prunes, but it will give you a boost of iron as well. If you couple this with a cup of chicory coffee, or a warm drink like herbal tea, it helps to soften and rehydrate poop that may be hard.

• Make sure that you are walking every day. Being too sedentary can slow your digestive system and bowels and not promote pooping.

• Reduce stress – incorporate self-care techniques to relax your digestive system.

• Take an **Emergen-C vitamin C packet** if your stomach is not sensitive to Vitamin C. Emergen-C vitamin C packets can be found in most grocery, drug and big box stores. It's a great way to jazz up your water and get your vitamin C, which is great for your digestive system, and the vitamin C promotes easy pooping.

• Digestive Enzyme—The one that we prefer is by **Kyolic™ Candida Cleanse & Digestion Formula 102**. It contains garlic and digestive enzymes to help get your digestive system back on track. Take 1-3 capsules after lunch and dinner with a glass of water.

• **Choose <u>one</u> type of magnesium**—See below. *Do not take both versions* or you will end up with severe diarrhea.

• **Natural Calm by Natural Vitality®**—Before bedtime, stir up a cup – cold or hot of Natural Calm by Natural Vitality®. It contains a proprietary blend of magnesium carbonate and citric acid. Once you add it to water, a chemical reaction binds the two together and creates ionic magnesium citrate. The Natural Calm product is not marketed as a laxative, but this magnesium supplement has a stool-softening side effect. The directions instruct users to decrease if loose stools occur (if you do not want this effect). But our family uses about 1 well-rounded teaspoon of the powder in a glass of water, and it keeps our family regular. You can adjust the serving amount to what works in producing a comfortable poop for you. Another wonderful perk of Natural Calm is it also promotes the most wonderful, restful, stress-free sleep.

OR

• **Natures Made® Magnesium Soft Gels**—If you do not have access to the above Natural Calm by Natural Vitality® magnesium or you would rather take a soft gel instead of drinking your magnesium, try Nature Made® Magnesium Soft Gels 250 mg per softgel. Nature Made® brands can be found in most drug, grocery and big box stores. It is very economical and easy to purchase. I recommend taking 2 softgels at nighttime with a glass of water. Please make sure that it is the 250 mg per softgel version. If you can't find the 250 mg, you may take <u>one</u> 400 mg softgel instead.

Choose <u>One</u> Type of Oil Supplement to Take—Do Not Take Both Oils

• **Nature Made® Flaxseed Oil Soft Gels 1400 mg**—Take one capsule right before bed with your magnesium supplement. The omega-3 fatty acids contained in the oil are a plant-based source of omega-3 and can help support heart health as well as help to soften any poop in your system.

<u>OR</u>

• **KYOLIC® Omega 3 Fish Oil Formula**—Take one capsule right before bed with your magnesium supplement. **KYOLIC® Omega-3** is a molecularly distilled fish oil concentrate, quality tested for heavy metals and PCB's for maximum purity and potency, providing one of the purest and richest levels of sustainable omega-3 essential fatty acids, EPA and DHA. This highly purified and concentrated fish oil is sourced from the cold, pristine waters of Norway. It is then combined with odorless Aged Garlic

Extract™. Fish oil also supports healthy circulation in the body and a natural anti-inflammatory response.

If you have been taking commercial laxatives you may have to wean yourself from taking them. Gradually take slightly less each week until you don't need to take the laxative. This gradual process of elimination will help to get your bowels back to working on their own, instead of depending upon a laxative to get them going. Please don't go cold turkey and forego the laxative. Your body will need some time to re-learn that it can poop on its own.

Do include a cup of coffee in the morning. The coffee caffeine does some wonderful work! It can activate contractions in your colon and intestinal muscles. Contractions in the colon help to push the contents of your bowels towards the rectum, producing the pooping sensation.

CHAPTER 24: CONSTIPATION DURING CHEMOTHERAPY

When I received the diagnosis that I had cancer and needed chemotherapy, the first thing that popped into my mind was, 'My hair will fall out, and I'm scared. I don't want to be nauseous and throwing up all the time." Not once did I think that constipation would be a big problem. Well, it is a big problem because of the medications that are administered before, during, and after to reduce pain, tolerate chemotherapy, and reduce nausea can cause constipation. Between the pain medications, anxiety medications, acid reducers, antihistamines, and the chemotherapy and immunity boosters, the body will have a difficult time producing a bowel movement. Most of the above medications slow the digestive tract down and anesthetize the nerves and muscle response in the body. It takes a few days before things return to somewhat "normal" function in the digestive tract, so you get the sensation that you feel like pooping again. The best tactic is to be as proactive as possible before, during, and after chemotherapy to assure that your digestive system is comfortable and functioning as well as possible.

The evening before chemotherapy, I would take 2 soft gels 250 mg each of Nature's Made Magnesium supplements, 1 tablet senna, 1 flaxseed supplement, and drink ½ cup of prune juice. I would repeat this every evening for 4-5 nights. I usually did not poop the day after chemotherapy. The first time, it kind of freaked me out, because I could not get the sensation to go, but I felt like I had to. But later I realized that all of the medications were causing my system to be somewhat numb. So of course, the sensation to go was just not going to happen. The next day it got better, and I finally went. It was a little bit of a struggle as nerve and muscle response is not fully engaged at that point. But it did get better with each day that passed.

New Chapter® SuperCritical Omega 7—I started taking this product before I developed cancer and had to go through chemotherapy. I initially took it because it was helpful when I occasionally had bouts with GERD (acid reflux). The omega 7 took care of my acid reflux in a matter of a few days, so I did not have to take acid reducers daily for GERD. Incidentally, the omega 7 also gave me improved skin tone—my skin a great glow.

I remembered how helpful the omega 7 was for my GERD, so I experimented to see if it would be helpful for chemotherapy nausea. I discovered that it was helpful for nausea and helped the digestive tract to repair itself after the chemotherapy treatment.

I took two capsules right before breakfast, 2 capsules before lunch, and 2 more capsules two hours after dinner.

I also took the omega 7 in conjunction with acid reducers first thing in the morning. It helped to decrease the nausea time and helped me return to being able to eat. I really like that it is a 100% vegetarian source of omega fatty acids made with organic sea buckthorn extract combined with rosemary and calendula. I have tried other Omega 7 products, and this one seems to make a big difference and work the best for nausea and digestive tract rebuilding.

Nature Made® Magnesium Soft Gels

Nature Made® Magnesium Soft Gels 250 mg per softgel. Nature Made brand can be found in most drug, grocery and big box stores. It is very economical and very easy to purchase. I recommend taking 2 softgels (250 mg each) at nighttime with a glass of water.

My Oncologist asked me how my constipation was going, and I told her about my magnesium find. She then replied, "Oh, that is good to hear! Magnesium is also very good for the heart, so this is great not only for constipation, but also heart health." So, if you are getting chemotherapy, magnesium sounds like a good way to keep pooping easily and to keep your heart healthy during the stress and strain of chemotherapy.

Natures Made® Flaxseed Oil Soft Gels 1400 mg—Take one capsule right before bed with your magnesium supplement. When you take flaxseed oil, the omega-3 fatty acids contained in the oil are a plant-based source of omega-3 and can help to support heart health.

Senna—I was a little hesitant to add Senna to my chemotherapy pooping plan. I had used it occasionally in the past, and it had given me cramping and an intense pooping sensation. Very uncomfortable. But when going through chemotherapy, it was a whole different story! It really was the perfect ticket to producing the pooping sensation when my body was dealing with so many medications that over-relaxed the digestive muscles and nerve reactions, making pooping impossible. I highly recommend it, but please check with your physicians to make sure it is appropriate for your treatment plan.

Please note: Senna can be added if you are not sensitive to senna or have an allergy.

Consult with your physician to make sure senna is safe for you.

If you have had a bowel obstruction, ulcerative colitis, Crohn's disease, appendicitis, or any digestive tract cancer, do not use it before consulting a physician.

Prune Juice—1/2–1 glass of prune juice at bedtime. Some people warm the prune juice in the microwave prior to drinking to "enhance" its poop-promoting properties. I have not done this. I have also heard that some nurses will suggest putting 1 tsp of butter into the prune juice before warming to really enhance the prune juice poop-promoting action. Either way, after reading a lot of blogs and chat boards, the unanimous vote was...definitely include prune juice.

CHAPTER 25: CONCLUSION

When I came up with the concept of writing this book, I hesitated. I mean, who writes a book about pooping? It seemed kind of well... uncomfortable, embarrassing, and an unconventional subject to embark upon. It's such a personal subject, but when I googled and saw the statistics of how many people had problems pooping, including my own family. I knew I had to write this embarrassing and personally uncomfortable book.

I really hope that the tips and suggestions in this book will help you, your family, or a loved one. And I truly hope that the tips and suggestions in the book will work for you. I want you to realize that it may take some time to help your body get back to pooping on its own. Not everyone will be able to achieve pooping naturally and effortlessly right away. It may take some time to undo the years of not doing the right things that your body needs to poop. So please understand, this book will not guarantee 100% success for everyone, especially not right out of the gate. After all, your body may need to relearn and get into a new routine.

Start out implementing as many suggestions as feels comfortable for you, then add more each week or month. And of course, it all depends upon your individual health and wellness. But please implement as many suggestions as you can; it can only help you move towards better health. Even if you implement 1-2 suggestions per month, by the end of the year, you will feel better and perhaps be closer to pooping on your own. Always check with your physician or health professional prior to trying anything new in your daily routine. I wish you all love, happiness and health always –Inci Jones

RESOURCE SECTION:

Supplements:

Bean-o®: available on Amazon, CVS, Target, and most drug or chain stores

Natural Calm® by Natural Vitality: AllStarHealth.com

Metamucil® : available on Amazon, CVS, Target, and most drug or chain stores

Probiotics—Suggested Brands: **PB8®, Nature's Way®, Kyo-Dophilus® by Kyolic, Ultra Jarrow Dophilus®**: AllStarHealth.com

Fish Oil: **Kyolic® Omega 3 Fish Oil Formula**

Protein Shake—**Orgain® Plant Protein Shake**: Available at Costco, AllStarHealth.com

Emergen-C® Packets: Available at Costco and AllStarHealth.com

Kyolic® Candida Cleanse & Digestion Formula 102: All Star Health.com

Nature's Made®—Magnesium Soft Gels in 250 mg or 400 mg: Costco, Target, CVS, Rite-Aid, or most drug chains

Nature's Made®—Flaxseed Oil Soft Gels Costco, Target, CVS, Rite-Aid, or most drug chains

New Chapter®—SuperCritical Omega 7: Amazon, AllStarHealth.com , CVS

Senna—I've used **Senokot**® (from the drug store) and **Nature's Way**® **Senna** (health food store) and both seem to work the same.

Food & Beverages

Ezekiel® **Bread:** available at most grocery stores.

Chicory Coffee

Bone Broth

Coconut Oil

Grass-Fed Meat

Prune Juice

Useful Household Items:

Bread Machine – **Zojirushi**® Bread Maker –

Printed in Dunstable, United Kingdom

70453934R00061

HELP GOING POOP

A WOMAN'S GUIDE TO GOING #2 NATURALLY
COMBAT CONSTIPATION WITHOUT LAXATIVES

INCI JONES

Abundant health & happiness.

Inci